BE YOUNG
WITH YOGA

RICHARD L. HITTLEMAN

PRENTICE-HALL, INC.

ENGLEWOOD CLIFFS, N. J.

PHOTOS BY EDWARD A. BOLLINGER

North Miami Beach, Florida

This book is dedicated to all those
students whose patient practice and
detailed reports through the years were
of such great assistance in the preparation of this work.

FOREWORD

You may undertake the practice outlined in this book almost regardless of your age or physical background. You are not to be concerned with how "stiff" or "out of condition" you think you are or whether you will be "able to do" the Yoga techniques. The reason you are going to practice Yoga is because you very probably *are* out of condition and Yoga works out stiffness, tension, tightness, flabbiness and many other negative conditions which sap your energy and health and prevent you from living a full life. Concerning whether you will be able to do these exercises, I will tell you that I have personally taught these movements to thousands of students and have never yet met a person who cannot do enough Yoga to experience great benefits almost at once. This is true of students 80 years of age and beyond as well as people of all ages who have allowed themselves to deteriorate into poor physical condition from lack of the proper physical activity.

Yoga is not 'exercise' in the ordinary sense of the word with strain, exertion, many repetitions and quick movements. In Yoga we conserve our energy, we should never experience any strain, only several repetitions are necessary and we do almost everything in slow-motion! There is nothing scientific about ordinary exercising. Only certain parts of the body are exercised in a 'hit' and 'miss' fashion. Some muscles will be used, some areas may be stretched and strengthened. But most 'key' areas of tension, strain and weakness will not receive any serious attention. The movements of Yoga, however, are able to stimulate and relax every part of the body from the toes to the scalp and from the muscles and tendons inward to the deepest internal organs and glands. This is why "20 minutes of Yoga is worth hours of ordinary exercise."

If you are ill or have a history of illness and you are in doubt as to how any of these postures may apply to your personal condition, *you must always consult your physician.* Show him the illustrations of this book. He is the only person qualified to tell you the kind of exercise you may undertake. My experience has been that physicians are generally eager to have their patients remain active and the mildness of the Yoga movements makes them particularly advantageous for those who want to keep fit and trim without strain and using the least amount of energy.

By following the simple instructions exactly as presented to you in this book, you will experience wonderful results in a short period of time. After a few weeks of practice you will come to realize that you are engaged in the most complete, well-thought-out system of physical health that has ever been devised. And the way you are going to *look* and *feel* will be the proof!

Richard L. Hittleman

Los Angeles, California
November, 1961

INTRODUCTION

Eternal Youth—Fiction or Fact?

Since time began, man has sought the fountain of youth. It has always been his dream to remain perpetually young. In history, legend and fable we read of his eternal quest for the magic formula that will roll back the years and restore to him the wonderful attributes of youth. And at some time during our lives we all wonder, "Is it really possible to become young again?"

To cater to this desire for youthfulness, our attention is continually called to a 'wonder' hormone that will return your vitality; to a 'new' skin cream with 'incredible acting' ingredients; to a 'miracle' formula which will "take years off your life", or to a marvelous machine which will do all the 'streamlining' without any effort on your part. And although most people who buy and try these 'miracle' products do so with tongue in cheek, the fact that millions of dollars are spent each year on just such things is conclusive evidence that man (and of course, woman) will never abandon the search for his lost youth.

Efforts along these lines are natural, for youth is synonymous with so many of the things which make life rich and enjoyable, —vigor, vitality, optimism and probably most important of all, lack of illness and disease; in other words HEALTH. But I ask you to consider for a moment the possibility that these tremendous efforts to hold back the years may be completely misdirected and that the reason we have not found a satisfactory solution to the problems of 'aging' is because *we have been looking in the wrong direction.*

There is an ancient Hindu legend of a warrior who roamed the entire world in search of a precious stone which he had lost. After a fruitless journey of many years, he returned to his home village, only to have a child point out to him that the very stone which he sought in distant lands was imbedded in his own forehead!

By the same token, I should like you to consider that the treasure of youth cannot be found on the *outside* no matter how far you travel and where you search. *The secret is within you!* In order to discover it you must now turn your attention inward. You have only to learn and experience a few simple laws of nature and you will do more to restore and maintain the wonderful characteristics of youth within 7 weeks than you could with all of the self-improvement fads, machines, devices, formulae and gadgets which have ever appeared.

The Real Meaning of 'Youth' and 'Age'

Let us see if we can catch a glimpse of this elusive thing called 'youth' so that we may know better what it is we are searching for.

When you speak about being 'young' or 'old' you are usually not referring to a definite age in terms of years but rather to a state of body and mind. If you stop to think for a moment you will realize that how 'young' a person looks and feels has nothing to do with his actual age in years, for one man is 'youthful' at 75 while another is 'old' at 40. What is the difference between these two individuals? It is simple. There are obvious *characteristics* which enable us to tell almost at a glance if a person is young or old. The more characteristics of youth that a person has, the more 'youthful' he or she *looks* and *feels* and *is*. The youthful man who is 75 has retained the characteristics of youth. Consequently he is vibrant and alive. The man who is old at 40 has lost the characteristics of youth and has acquired many or all of the symptoms of age. He therefore appears 'old'.

What are these characteristics of youth? What are the characteristics of age? Let us list the 8 major ones which will concern us in this book.

YOUTH	AGE
1. Flexibility—suppleness—agility; grace—poise—balance.	Stiffness—tightness—immobility; awkwardness—lack of poise.
2. Ability to relax as necessary—calmness—composure—serenity; restful sleep.	Tension—nervousness—irritability—poor disposition; insomnia.
3. Vitality—energy—endurance.	Fatigue — weariness — exhaustion.
4. Proper blood circulation resulting in the health and strength of vital organs and glands.	Inadequate blood circulation with resultant dull complexion, wrinkles, general poor health.
5. Resilience of muscles resulting in firmness, taut skin; strength.	Loss of muscle tone resulting in weakness, sagging and flabbiness.

YOUTH	AGE
6. Normal weight (in accordance with bone structure) and ability to control and correctly distribute weight.	Obesity; inability to control and maintain correct weight.
7. Quick replacement of vital elements continually used by body and brain.	Slowness or loss of ability to replace these vital elements.
8. Alertness and clarity of the faculties of mind; optimism.	Weakening of the faculties of mind resulting in senility; depression.

Consider each of these 'youth' characteristics carefully and you will realize that whatever you have lost on the 'youth' side you are in the process of gaining on the 'age' side.

The Wrong Approach to the Problems of 'Aging'

Now it may appear to be a tremendous task to regain these 'youth' characteristics. But this is true only because you are probably accustomed to dealing with each of these vital factors through a *different* machine, a *different* pill or a *different* device. For example, you may take a tonic for your blood, a tranquilizer for your nerves, have a massage to work out the stiffness in your back, go to the gym to keep your muscles firm, undertake a diet to control your weight, etc. The point is that most people not only believe that they must cope with the 'age' symptoms through many different devices which are found outside of themselves (such as the tonics, the machines, the massages) but that these devices are somehow or other going to result in a permanent solution to their problems. These beliefs are false. And because the principle upon which the devices are founded is erroneous people are forever on the lookout for a new pill, machine or gadget to give them the help they are seeking.

Take for example the problem of excess weight which so plagues Americans today and is probably responsible for many of our illnesses. When you find yourself getting the beginnings of a 'bay window' and growing heavy in the arms and thighs, you naturally put off doing anything about it as long as you possibly can. But there comes the day of reckoning when you run out of excuses and postponements and you know that something must be done. You are faced with a number of choices: go to the gym and 'work it off' (a most unpleasant prospect); start counting calories and go on one of the numerous 'miracle' reducing plans (which somehow seem to work out miraculously for the people in the advertisement but never quite give you the same results); or finally get yourself a machine with all the gadgets that will do the work for you so that all you have to do is lie back and allow the machine to 'rub away that ugly fat'. This last choice is generally the most appealing. Who, in our day, wants to walk if they can ride?

Now using the gadgets of this machine for 'spot' and overall reducing is certainly the easy way out and it may even work until you realize one day that you are going to have to use this machine or gadget for the rest of your life because the moment you stop, back comes the excess weight. You will then find to your dismay that the same thing is true with steam baths, massages, diets, appetite deterrents, setting-up exercises, etc. They are all fine and may help you for as long as you use them. But as soon as you stop, the weight which has been lurking in the background all the time, comfortably returns home. Can you see why this is true? It is because you have never pierced through to the heart of the matter. *You have been dealing with the symptoms, not the cause.*

When there is a hole in the roof of your house and the water is leaking in, a temporary device is to catch the water in a bucket and empty the bucket each time it becomes full. But if you wanted a solution for the problem, you would repair the roof. The hole in the roof is the real trouble, not the water. By the same token, rubbing, steaming, dieting off excess weight is a temporary aid just like emptying the bucket. You are only coping with the symptoms. The same is true for the problems of tension, nervousness, fatigue, insomnia, stiffness, tightness, etc. If you want a solution for these physical problems you must deal directly with their causes.

The Cause and Solution for 'Age'

What are these causes? Well, let us carry this line of reasoning one step further. Haven't you wondered about why you may show the symptoms of age (often very prematurely) even though you seem to be doing all the necessary things to ward off the toll of the years? For example, why are you stiff and tight in vital areas of the body although you play 18 holes of golf, walk 3 miles and swim 10 times around the pool? Why do you lose your youthful vitality even though you are taking a multitude of 'energy' and 'pep' potions? Why can't you relax even though there is a bottle of tranquilizers always handy in your pocket? Why is your hair falling out in spite of the fact that you rub a generous quantity of the new 'X-436 Miracle Hair Tonic' into your scalp each day? Why do you get middle-age spread even though you do all the housework, shopping, gardening and feel you are extremely 'active'?

If we had to find a separate cause and a separate solution for each of these problems of remaining physically fit and youthful, the task would probably prove hopeless. But let me now ask this question: is it possible that lack of vitality, nervousness and tension, poor blood circulation, excess weight, stiffness, loss of muscle tone and even a weakening of the faculties of mind can all be attributed to *one cause* and that there is *one solution* for this cause? Our answer is, *positively, yes!* Here is the *cause* for the symptoms of age:

IMPROPER CARE OF THE BODY

Here is the *solution* to the problem:

KNOWLEDGE OF CORRECT CARE FOR THE BODY
This knowledge consists of the following four principles:

1. There lies *within* you (*and only within you*) the tremendous vital force necessary to continually regenerate your physical organism.

2. This vital force permeates every atom of your being and is extremely active in the early years of your life. But unless it is periodically stimulated and activated, it will become less active and more dormant as the years go by. It does not disappear. It just gradually goes to sleep.

3. Only *you* through your own efforts are capable of truly awakening and stimulating this dormant vital force once again.

4. This awakening is accomplished by manipulating your body in such a manner that organs, glands, nerves, cells, bones and joints where the vital force lies asleep is methodically stimulated, nourished, stretched and relaxed.

We may summarize the above by stating that the major causes and symptoms of 'aging' are due to not caring properly for the body. The greatest part of this improper care lies in not knowing the type of activity necessary to activate the vital force of regeneration. We have already seen how a person may be extremely 'active' and still gain weight and become stiff. This person generally thinks of being 'active' in terms of how much movement he makes or how much energy he uses up. He does not understand that simply movement and energy are of little value. It is the *type* of movement that is important. Therefore, it is possible to prevent loss of muscle tone by knowing what *type* of movements are necessary to strengthen every area of the body. You can relieve tension, nervous strain and stiffness by knowing what *type* of movements truly relax the body. Only the *type* of activity will restore the youthful characteristics to you. This is the whole secret.

Question: where do you get the machine or apparatus that provides the correct activity?

Answer: you look for no help from the outside. You employ no machines or apparatus of any kind. You accomplish your goal entirely by yourself through the world's oldest and most respected science of reconditioning and developing— *physical (Hatha) Yoga.*

The World's Oldest Science of Remaining Youthful

A 'Yogi' is a person who practices Yoga. The Yogi considers 'old-age' as we know it, to be unnatural! To him, atrophication of the body and brain is not 'inevitable' just because one grows older in years.

Is it the natural state of man to be stiff, weak, exhausted, tense, nervous, depressed, overweight; to lose vitality, endurance and the faculties of his mind; to be subject to an infinite number of illnesses and diseases which leave him deformed, withered, stooped, shrunken and wracked with pain? Is it natural to be deprived of the ability to live a fulfilled life? The Yogi's answer is an emphatic "no!" He has been most successful in proving his point.

The science of Yoga is becoming known to an ever increasing number of health-minded persons throughout the world who have bought and tried the multitude of health and youth products, only to meet with one disappointment after another.

If you were in the market for a particular product, and you learned that there was a company selling this product who had been in business for some 3,000 years with sales increasing continually, you would certainly be impressed by this phenomenal record. If, upon further investigation into this company, you found that thousands of competitors who had attempted to market a similar product had all, sooner or later, gone out of business, there would be no doubt in your mind as to the superiority of the company which had endured these many centuries.

We have exactly this situation when we speak of Yoga. It is of such great age that its history is lost in dim antiquity and yet, long after the currently popular imitation physical health fads and mental development methods have faded away and new ones have come and gone (as they do more and more quickly) Yoga will prevail. This is because Yoga is the original in its field; it has been perfected over a period of countless centuries and it always works!

The Importance of Yoga for Americans

Americans can now profit enormously from Yoga, once they learn how enjoyable it is to practice, and the remarkable benefits which can result from doing this form of exercise only a few minutes each day.

The incredible misconceptions that new students often have when they come to me for the first time to inquire about Yoga are indeed astonishing. These misconceptions range from the young man who wondered if the catcher for the New York Yankees studied with us to the elderly lady who informed me that she would love to try Yoga but she thought that her skin was too delicate to sit on the bed of nails for more than a few seconds at a time. I could probably write an entire book of humorous anecdotes regarding such misconceptions. But in another sense, the ideas concerning Yoga which so many people have acquired through completely misinformed sources is an extremely tragic affair, for the very thing which Americans so desperately need today is health,—the knowledge of how to care for their bodies and minds, and the simple practice of Yoga will go further toward regaining and maintaining health and youth than any other physical activity in which we engage for this purpose!

Who Can Practice Yoga?

Although we have already spoken briefly about this, it is important to note again that neither age nor physical condition is a barrier in this practice. The more 'out of condition', 'stiff', 'weak', 'tense', 'irritable' that you are, the more you need the movements and postures of Yoga. Wherever you are tense, stiff, weak, etc. is where your vitality and energy are being drained and where future maladies can strike. Such conditions never become better by being ignored. They always become worse. I have explained about consulting your physician in the event that you have or have had an illness and you are not sure as to how these techniques may apply.

Two or more members of a family who have taken our class course often practice together at home. If you can seriously interest the members of your family in this work you will find you have done them a great service. Naturally, the youngsters will generally be able to assume the postures more quickly because they are flexible (one of the characteristics of youth). But don't let them embarrass you with their agility. With a little practice you will find yourself becoming as young as they in flexibility. It is interesting and important to note here that many children have become interested in Yoga because they have seen their parents practicing at home. Children love to move their bodies in the positions of the Yoga postures and if you can start them off with these techniques while they are young in years they will be eternally grateful. Once they establish the patterns of Yoga they will never give it up. Also, remember that Yoga does not excite; it calms. Therefore it often proves extremely beneficial for nervous children.

It does not matter if one person cannot go as far as the next in these postures. Each physical organism is as individual as its owner and the histories and conditions of no two bodies are the same. You are in competition with no one in the practice of Yoga. Therefore, it does not matter how well you are able to perform these techniques in the beginning because you will receive the full benefit according to your particular structure.

What You Need to Practice Yoga

1. Learn and practice your postures in a quiet place with the least number of distractions.

2. You need only sufficient room to stretch out on a flat surface. This surface should be covered by a blanket, towel, straw mat, rug or mattress pad.

3. A watch or clock with an easily-read second hand will prove helpful.

4. Dress in any comfortable clothing which provides freedom for your body and enables you to stretch. Shorts, slacks, leotards, gym clothing is satisfactory. Anything tight or confining about your body such as shoes, belt, watch, eyeglasses should be removed.

5. Make certain that there is a plentiful supply of fresh air in the place where you are practicing.

6. I should like to suggest that you do not idly exhibit as a curiosity or talk about your Yoga practice except to persons who you feel are sincerely interested. You will lose a great deal of the power of Yoga by treating it lightly.

When Do You Practice?

You need approximately 20 to 40 minutes which can be divided up over the day as necessary. You will receive detailed instructions regarding this in the text of the book. This 20 to 40 minutes is an excellent investment because the returns and dividends both in enjoyment and efficiency cannot be duplicated through any other physical means. You can practice *before* eating, as you wish, but always wait at least 90 minutes *after* a meal to begin your practice. You may find it interesting to learn that many of our business and professional men who have taken my class course take a few minutes out during a 'break' in the day's work to revitalize and refresh themselves through several simple techniques which may be used for this purpose. You will learn these extremely practical techniques in this book. There are executives who will not engage in activities such as business conferences which require particular clarity and alertness of mind unless they have first prepared themselves through certain of these techniques. This may seem a bit far-fetched to you at this point but after your first two or three weeks of practice, it will no longer seem unusual. You will have a great insight into the force and power which is generated through this practice.

To emphasize the fact that Yoga can be practiced at many times during the day I should like to tell you that you will find you have a wonderful weapon against fatigue and depression. This is true for the housewife who finds herself tense, stiff and tired from the chores of her housework as well as for the businessman who comes home at night, exhausted. If instead of collapsing in your chair or lying down for a nap you will go through 20 minutes of Yoga practice, you will find that stiffness and tension are removed as if by magic and that you get your 'second wind'. It is important to point out here that Yoga is the only system of physical culture which deals simultaneously with relaxation of the mind. In other words, by doing the physical movements you will find that you are greatly relaxed not only in body *but also in mind*. You have only to test this program a few times to experience the results.

The Results You Can Expect

By practicing the 20 techniques exactly as taught to you in this book, you can expect to accomplish the following:

1. Strengthen and recondition your entire body.
2. Regain youthful flexibility in spine and limbs.
3. Help control and redistribute your weight in accordance with your physical structure.
4. Remove tension from its many hiding places in your body.
5. Remain relaxed under pressure.
6. Store and release energy and vital force to be used as needed.
7. Heighten resistance to many common disorders.
8. Restore grace, balance, poise and self-confidence.
9. Awaken the vital force to help gain control of your emotions and your mind.
10. Improve in every one of your activities.

You now have read all of the material necessary to begin your practice. In this book I do not intend to present a history of the various types of Yoga, replete with Sanskrit terms. What is needed here is for you simply to experience the remarkable new lease on life which the contents of this book have to offer. With each week we will trade more of the characteristics of age for the characteristics of youth by reawakening the elements of youth which have gone to sleep within you. When a light is turned on, the darkness vanishes. As you regain youth, age disappears.

So resolve now that you will allow nothing to interfere with your next 7 weeks of Yoga practice and let's begin!

HOW TO USE
THIS BOOK

Part I of this text contains the instructions and information for learning 20 dynamic Yoga techniques in a 7 week plan. You will find each of the techniques presented in the following outline:

What the Technique Does for You

Under this heading you will find a list of the benefits that you can expect to derive from each technique if you practice as advised.

How To Do the Technique

The information here consists of a group of simple steps for learning how to do each technique. Carefully read the entire method first; study the illustrations; lay the book down near you where you may refer to it as necessary. Try the exercise. Repeat the movements several times to make sure that you have learned the exercise correctly. When you understand how the technique is performed, proceed to the next exercise of that week.

How to Practice the Technique

Here you are advised of the period of time to hold the posture; the number of repetitions and the best time of the day to practice that particular technique. It is essential that you practice according to the time advised for each exercise. Therefore you must keep your mind on your counting. Most of the techniques are done in *seconds*. It is simple to count approximate seconds silently to yourself. Try it with your watch a few times to get the feel of 10, 15 and 20 seconds. You will need to use your watch only a few times in this work.

It is best to do some of these exercises in the morning (designated in the text as AM) and others in afternoon, evening or at night (PM). This is also indicated for you with each technique. It is not essential that you do them exactly as specified if your time or schedule does not permit. You may have to modify the program somewhat. However, try to follow the suggestions as closely as possible.

Important Things You Will Want To Know About the Technique

Under this heading you will find interesting and important information about each technique which you will want to consider.

Points to Remember When Practicing the Technique

The information here consists of refinements which will prove helpful for getting the most from your practice.

Weekly Plan of Practice

You are instructed in a simple step-by-step method through-out this 7 week plan. After you learn the new exercises on the first two days of each week you are referred to the WEEKLY PLAN OF PRACTICE at the end of that section. When you have completed the 7 weeks of study you will then use the COMPLETE PLAN OF PRACTICE which appears at the end of Part I.

Part II of this book goes into detail regarding each of the characteristics of youth as outlined on page 5 and indicates certain of the 20 techniques which can be emphasized for specific problems. Although the text of Part II can be read in conjunction with Part I you should complete the seven weeks of practice and perform the COMPLETE PLAN OF PRACTICE for at least four weeks exactly as indicated before you devote additional practice time to the special routines listed in Part II.

CONTENTS

Part II

BE YOUNG
WITH YOGA

Part I

YOGA IN 7 WEEKS

FIRST WEEK

On the first and second days of this First Week carefully learn the 6 techniques listed below. During these 2 days devote as much time as you can to learning.

1. PRELIMINARY LEG PULL
2. KNEE AND THIGH STRETCH
3. BACKWARD BEND
4. TOE TWIST
5. ARM AND LEG STRETCH
6. LOTUS POSTURES

On the 3rd day of this week turn to page 58 and practice according to the 'Practice Plan' for the remainder of this first week.

YOUTH

through *STRETCHING THE LEGS AND LOOSENING THE SPINE CONCAVELY*

● Technique No. 1—PRELIMINARY LEG PULL

What the Preliminary Leg Pull Does for You

1. Removes stiffness and promotes elasticity in the spine through a *concave* stretching movement.

2. Helps to relieve tension in the back.

3. Stretches and strengthens the entire leg.

4. Makes the muscles and skin of the legs taut and firm.

How To Do the Preliminary Leg Pull

1. Sit on the floor with your legs extended straight out in front of you, feet together and backs of the knees touching the floor.

2. Extend your arms straight out in front of you so that your hands are at eye level.

3. *Very slowly* stretch as far forward as you can and aim your hands for the farthermost part of your legs.

4. Grasp the farthermost part of your legs that you can hold without strain. This may be the knee, calf, ankle, foot or toe. (Fig. 1)

5. Gently, in *slow motion*, bend your elbows outward and pull yourself forward and downward until you reach the point beyond which you can no longer stretch comfortably. Stop wherever this movement becomes difficult,

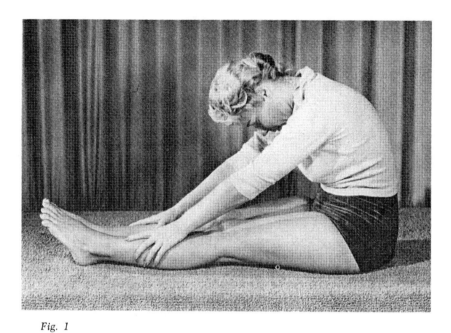

Fig. 1

Subject is Miss Eve Diskin, secretary, who has been practicing Yoga for approximately 18 months.

PHOTO CREDITS: Edward A. Bollinger, North Miami Beach, Florida

Fig. 2

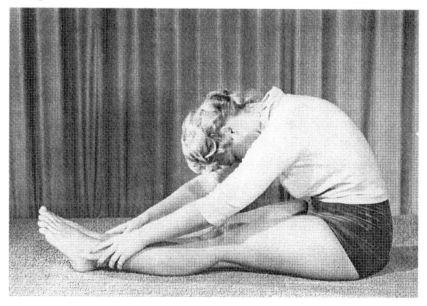

for there is never to be any strain in the practice of Yoga. Hold your extreme position absolutely motionless for the advised number of seconds. Do not fidget, fight or strain. (Fig. 2)

6. When the count is completed, *very slowly,* raise your trunk to the upright position. Rest easily for several moments and repeat as advised.

How To Practice the Preliminary Leg Pull

Time to hold the extreme
position: °   begin with 10 seconds; add
                       5 seconds weekly until you
                       reach 20 seconds.
Number of times: 3
Time of the day: AM and/or PM

Important Things To Know About the Preliminary Leg Pull

This technique will be an indication as to how stiff and tight you may have grown in 'Key' areas throughout your back and legs. The PRELIMINARY LEG PULL will begin to loosen these tense and cramped spots and provide you with elasticity of the spine. By following the directions exactly as given and holding your extreme position without motion for the number of seconds indicated, you will soon be able to place your forehead very close to, if not actually on your knees.

° We count the seconds or minutes *only for the extreme position,* not for any of the movements which lead into or out of the extreme position.

**Points To Remember When Practicing
the Preliminary Leg Pull**

1. Never strain. Go only as far as you are able to bend comfortably in slow motion and hold your extreme position motionless. Do not jerk or fight in order to get down a little farther. Each day you will find that your spine automatically gains in elasticity by following the above directions.

2. Make certain that the backs of both knees remain resting on the floor and that your legs are held straight.

3. Remember to bend your elbows slightly outward as you draw your head downward.

4. Count the necessary number of seconds silently to yourself. You may close your eyes if you wish.

YOUTH

for the *KNEES AND THIGHS*

● Technique No. 2—KNEE AND THIGH STRETCH

What the Knee and Thigh Stretch Does for You

1. Helps to remove stiffness and tension in the knees and thighs.

2. Enables you to walk and stand without becoming easily tired.

How To Do the Knee and Thigh Stretch

1. Extend your legs straight out before you.

2. Bend your legs at the knees and bring your feet in as far as possible toward you. Place the soles of the feet together.

3. Clasp your hands firmly around your feet. (Fig. 3)

4. Pull up on your feet with your hands and allow your knees and thighs to bend downward as far as possible without strain. Sit erectly and hold your extreme position for the advised number of seconds. Do not fidget, fight or strain. (Fig. 4)

5. Relax and allow the knees and thighs to return to the position of Fig. 3. Remain with your hands clasped around your feet so that you may repeat as advised.

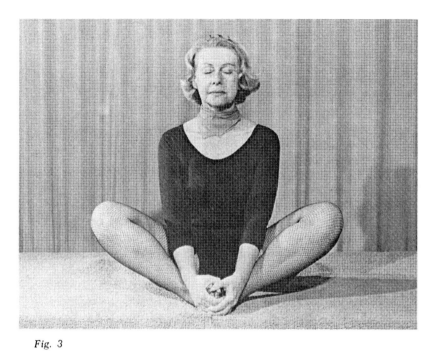

Fig. 3

Model for these photographs is Mrs. J. Goldbach, housewife, who has been practicing for 2 years.

Fig. 4

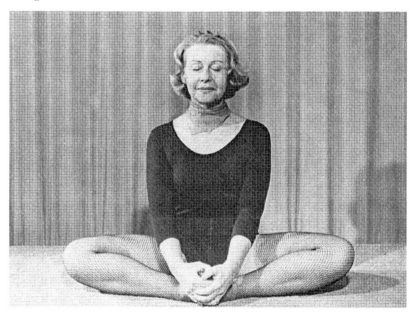

How To Practice the
Knee and Thigh Stretch

Time to hold the extreme position:	15 seconds
Number of times:	3
Time of the day:	AM and/or PM

Important Things To Know About the
Knee and Thigh Stretch

The major objective in this technique is to stretch out the seldom-exercised knees and thighs. You may find your knees quite some distance from the floor in the beginning. However, here again, with patience and practice they will gradually lower themselves toward the floor. It is of no consequence how *far* you are able to stretch in the beginning. The stretching itself is the important thing. As you continue to practice this technique, you will find that the "spring" returns to your legs and that you can walk and stand without becoming so easily tired. The YOGA stretching postures keep the joints limber and help to avert the painful bone and joint diseases which are characteristics of "old-age."

Points To Remember When Practicing
the Knee and Thigh Stretch

1. Sit erectly at all times. (There is a tendency to slump forward in this posture.)

2. Clasp your hands *firmly* around your feet.

3. Do not fight, jerk or strain to get the knees down an extra inch. You will make no progress through fighting. Simply remain in your extreme position *absolutely motionless* for the advised number of seconds. (Remember that this is true for all of the stretching techniques.)

4. Count the 15 seconds silently. You may close your eyes for relaxation.

YOUTH

**through STRENGTHENING THE
FEET AND LOOSENING THE
SPINE CONVEXLY**

● Technique No. 3—BACKWARD BEND

What the Backward Bend Does for You

1. Begins to promote elasticity in the spine through a *convex* (inward) stretching movement.

2. Helps to relieve tension throughout the spine.

3. Develops the chest and bust.

4. Strengthens the feet and toes.

How To Do the Backward Bend

1. Sit on your heels. The top of your feet are resting on the floor and your knees are together in front of you.

2. Place the palms of your hands so that they rest on the floor on either side of your body.   (Fig. 5)

3. Little by little, "walk" back with your hands until you reach a comfortable maximum.

4. Lower your head backward and push your abdomen and chest upward to form the greatest possible arch *without strain*. You must remain seated on your heels.   (Fig. 6) Remain in your extreme position for the advised number of seconds. Do not fidget, fight or strain. All extreme positions should be held motionless.

5. Relax by *slowly* lowering your abdomen and chest and raising your head. Try to stay seated on your heels and do not move your hands; the posture thus becomes easy to repeat.

6. To repeat, simply drop your head backward and push upward with your abdomen and chest as described in step 4.

7. To come out of the posture, *slowly* drop your abdomen and chest and raise your head; "walk" forward little by little until you are able to easily raise your trunk from your heels.

8. Change the position of your feet so that your toes now rest on the floor. (Fig. 7) If you are able to sit on your heels in this position, attempt to perform the exact movements of steps 2, 3 and 4 (above). Move very carefully and stop at whatever point this posture becomes uncomfortable. If this movement is uncomfortable for you, simply put as much weight as you can on your heels and toes and hold your position for the prescribed time.

9. Come out of the posture *very slowly* by "walking" forward little by little with your hands and fingers. Relax by sitting in a cross-legged posture. Massage your feet gently with your hands if necessary.

Fig. 5

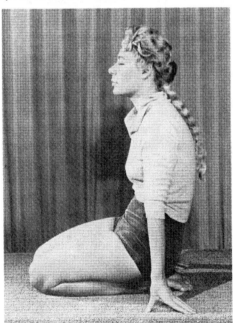

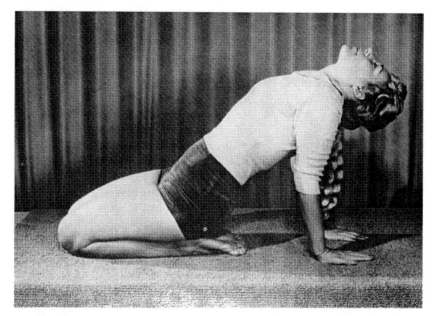

Fig. 6

Fig. 7

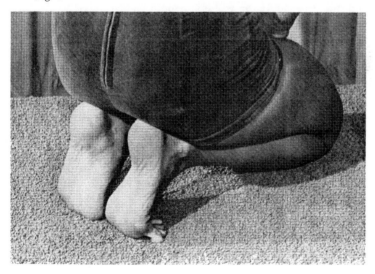

How To Practice the Backward Bend

Time to hold the 2 extreme positions:

begin with 10 seconds for both the foot and toe positions; add the seconds as advised in future weeks until 15 seconds are reached.

Number of times:

2 times on the feet
1 time on the toes

Time of the day:

AM and/or PM

Important Things To Know About the Backward Bend

In this technique, we will attempt to relieve tension through a *convex* (inward) stretching of the spine. Also, we will strengthen and gain elasticity in the feet and toes. You may experience some discomfort when you attempt to sit on your feet as instructed. This indicates that your feet have become weak and stiff and need to be gradually worked out and strengthened. If you will simply put as much weight as you can on your feet and patiently hold that position for the advised number of seconds, on the next day you will be able to support a little more weight. Within a few weeks you will certainly be able to rest the full body weight upon the feet. The same is true with the toes, although they are stubborn and usually require more time. I have never yet taught this posture to any student (including persons eighty years of age and beyond) who could not succeed with practice.

Points To Remember When Practicing the Backward Bend

1. Remain seated on your heels at all times during this movement.

2. Remember to drop your head backward. (We want the blood to run into the head.)

3. Keep your arms parallel with your sides and make sure your fingers point behind you. (See the illustrations in Fig. 5 and Fig. 6.)

4. Close your eyes and count the seconds silently.

5. Remember to come out of the posture by moving your palms forward little by little. Do not come lurching forward in a sudden movement.

YOUTH

through *STREAMLINING THE WAIST AND REGAINING BALANCE AND POISE*

● **Technique No. 4—TOE TWIST**

What the Toe Twist Does for You

1. Helps to remove stiffness and promote elasticity in the spine through a *spiral* stretching movement.

2. Aids in streamlining the abdominal area.

3. Strengthens the entire foot and leg.

4. Promotes balance, grace and poise.

How To Do the Toe Twist

1. Stand easily with your arms at your sides and your feet pointed slightly outward.

2. Raise your arms stiffly from your sides and stretch them straight out before you at eye level with the hands touching.

3. Raise your body up on your toes.   (Fig. 8)

4. Keeping your eyes fixed on the back of your hands turn the trunk *slowly* to the *left*. Go as far to your left as possible without strain, attempting to keep yourself balanced on your toes while your eyes gaze at the back of your hands.   (Fig. 9)   Hold your extreme position for the advised number of seconds.

5. Return *slowly* to the frontward position and *slowly* lower your arms to your sides. Stand easily for several moments without fidgeting or becoming restless. Execute the identical movements on the *right* side.

6. Return to the frontward position and repeat as advised.

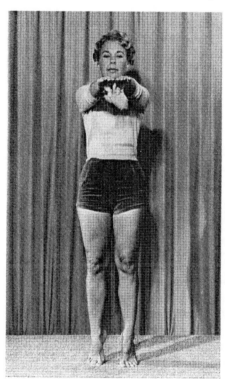

Fig. 8

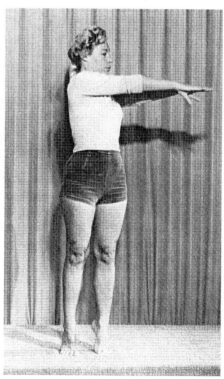

Fig. 9

How To Practice the Toe Twist

Time to hold the extreme position:	begin with 10 seconds; add the seconds as advised in future weeks until 20 seconds are reached.
Number of times:	2 times on either side. Begin with the left side, then go to the right. Repeat: left and right.
Time of the day:	AM and/or PM

Important Things To Know About the Toe Twist

Balance, grace and poise are important characteristics of youth and have a great effect on your appearance and your feeling of self-confidence. This technique will make you as graceful as a ballet dancer and at the same time will strengthen the entire leg through the slow turning to the sides while on the toes. Also, further elasticity of the spine is gained, this time through a *spiral* stretching movement. This spiral movement has a wonderful "streamlining" effect on the waist and often reduces excess weight in this abdominal area. You cannot expect to succeed in your first few attempts since remaining on the toes·is difficult. But within a week you should be well on your way toward regaining this highly important youthful characteristic: balance. You will sense a mastery over your body as you succeed.

Points To Remember When Practicing the Toe Twist

1. Keep your eyes on the back of your hands at all times during this technique.

2. Always stay as high on your toes as possible.

3. Hold your abdomen in and your chest out as you go around to the sides. Try to keep a perfect posture.

4. If you lose your balance at any point in this exercise, *do not laugh or show any signs of discouragement.* Simply come right back up at the point where you lost your balance and continue the exercise. When you maintain a serious attitude in this work your body will realize that you intend to become the master and will respond accordingly. The body, in many cases, is very much like a child and must be correctly disciplined.

YOUTH

through *RELEASING TRAPPED ENERGY*

● Technique No. 5—ARM AND LEG STRETCH

What the Arm and Leg Stretch Does for You

1. Provides an immediate relief of tension in "key" areas of the legs and back, helping to eliminate fatigue.

2. Promotes balance, grace and poise.

How To Do the Arm and Leg Stretch

1. Stand easily with your arms at your sides.

2. *Slowly* raise your right arm stiffly overhead.

3. Shift your full weight to your right leg.

4. Bend your left leg at the knee and hold your left foot with your left hand. You will have to balance yourself on your right leg. (Fig. 10)

5. *Slowly* bring your right hand back a few inches and simultaneously raise your left leg a few inches so that you feel a gentle stretch in your back. Drop your head slightly backward and look upward. (Fig. 11) Remain in this position for the advised number of seconds. If you experience very much difficulty in keeping your balance, you may rest the upraised arm against a wall. But don't be too anxious to use the wall until you have tried this for several days, as the balance is usually quickly regained.

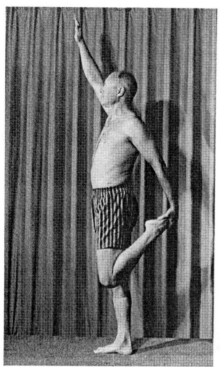

Fig. 10

Subject is Mr. Edward A. Bollinger, businessman, who has studied Yoga for 14 months.

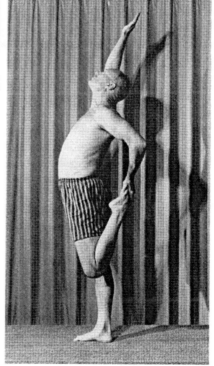

Fig. 11

6. *Slowly* lower your right arm to your side and your left foot to the floor. Stand easily for several moments and repeat as advised.

7. Perform the identical movements on the opposite side. Simply substitute the word "left" for "right" and vice-versa.

How To Practice the Arm and Leg Stretch

Time to hold the extreme position:	10 seconds
Number of times:	2 times on either side. Begin with your right arm and left leg; repeat. Change to your left am and right leg; repeat.
Time of the day:	AM and/or PM

Important Things To Know About the Arm and Leg Stretch

This is a wonderful technique to do at any time during the day when you need your "second wind." This type of *convex* stretch provides a quick relief of tension and releases trapped energy. The ARM AND LEG STRETCH works very intensely throughout the back. You will find that your spine is like a jack-in-the-box. It has been compressed into a small area through our ordinary sitting, working, driving and lying postures. The ARM AND LEG STRETCH is one of those techniques which open up the "box" and your spine is able to stretch out again, perhaps for the first time in many years. Whenever your spine becomes stiff, cramped and tense, you are bound to be sapped of your vitality. When you methodically stretch your spine you will regain your energy.

**Points To Remember When Practicing
the Arm and Leg Stretch**

1. This is another technique in which you will have to maintain your balance. If you experience real difficulty in doing this, you should rest the upraised arm against the wall.

2. Remember to drop your head slightly backward to add to the stretch. (See Fig. 11)

3. Keep your eyes open in this technique. Count the seconds silently. Concentrate carefully on what you are doing.

4. If you lose your balance, *do not laugh or show any signs of discouragement.* Compose yourself, come right back up and begin the count again. One week of practice should provide you with good control of this exercise.

YOUTH

through *RELAXATION*
THE ELEMENTARY SITTING POSITION

● **Technique No. 6a—HALF-LOTUS**

What the Half-Lotus Does for You

1. Relaxes the entire nervous system.

2. Loosens tension and stiffness in the ankles, knees and thighs.

3. Provides a comfortable sitting position for resting the mind (meditation). It has been used for this purpose since time immemorial.

How To Do the Half-Lotus

1. In a sitting position, stretch your legs straight out before you.

2. Bend your *left* leg at the knee and bring it toward you so that you can take hold of your left foot with both hands.

3. Place your left foot so that the sole rests against the inside of the right thigh. The heel of your left foot should be drawn in as far as possible.

4. Now bend your right leg at the knee so that you can take hold of your right foot with both hands.

5. Place your right foot in the fold of your left leg. Drop the right knee as far as possible toward the floor. Rest your hands on your knees. (Fig. 12) Sit in this position as advised.

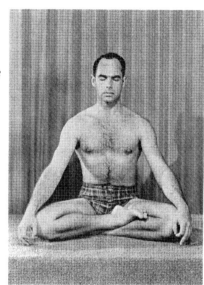

Fig. 12

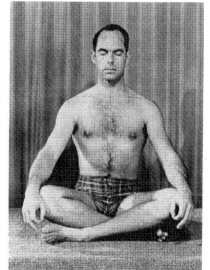

Fig. 13

Subject is Mr. Richard Leavitt, high
school instructor, who has practiced
Yoga for 2½ years.

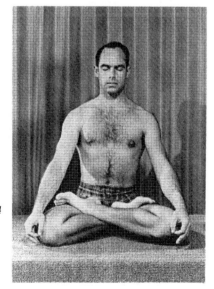

Fig. 14

6. When your legs grow tired, stretch them straight out before you and gently massage your knees. Then repeat the position by reversing the legs so that the *right* leg is drawn in first and the left leg is on top.

If the HALF-LOTUS posture as described above is too difficult for you, simply sit in the cross-legged posture of Fig. 13 and rest your forearms on your knees. Reverse the legs when necessary. By sitting in this easy posture, your knees will gradually lower themselves toward the floor and you will then be able to do the HALF-LOTUS.

YOUTH
through RELAXATION
THE ADVANCED SITTING POSITION

● Technique No. 6b—FULL-LOTUS

What the Full-Lotus Does for You

1. Provides the classical sitting position for resting the mind (meditation) during longer periods of time without bodily movement.

2. Promotes very great elasticity of the ankles, knees and legs because of the position which is required.

   The FULL-LOTUS is actually an advanced Yoga posture which generally requires practice and patience to accomplish. If you cannot do the HALF-LOTUS easily, you will be unable to assume the FULL-LOTUS.

   It is not necessary to attain the FULL-LOTUS in order to receive the full benefits of this course.

How To Do the Full-Lotus

1. In a sitting position, stretch your legs straight out before you.

2. Bend your *right* leg at the knee and bring it toward you so that you can take hold of your right foot with both hands.

3. Place your right foot on top of your left thigh. The right foot should be brought toward you as far as is possible so that eventually the right heel is touching the groin. In order to now complete the posture successfully, the right knee will have to rest on the floor.

4. Bend your left leg at the knee and bring it toward you so that you can take hold of your left foot with both hands.

5. Place your left foot on top of your right thigh. The left foot should be brought in as far as possible so that eventually the left heel will also touch the groin. Both knees should eventually rest on the floor. (Fig. 14) Sit in this position as advised.

6. When your legs grow tired, stretch them straight out before you and gently massage your knees. Then repeat the position by reversing the legs so that *left* leg is drawn in first and the right leg is on top. (It is usual to find the LOTUS postures more comfortable with one leg on top than the other due to the fact that the structure of the legs varies.)

How To Practice the Lotus Postures

Time to hold the extreme positions of the HALF-LOTUS, FULL-LOTUS or simple cross-legged postures: as long as possible without discomfort. (This varies greatly among students.) Reverse the legs as necessary.

Time of the day: whenever it is possible to relax in this manner.

Important Things To Know About the Lotus Postures

Sit in one of the LOTUS postures to read your newspaper, watch TV or relax your body and rest your mind. The LOTUS postures provide comfortable sitting positions in which you can remain for extended periods of time without continual adjustment of the trunk and legs. With practice you will find that you can sit in this fashion for 20 minutes and longer. The flexibility which is required in the legs is quickly gained and this flexibility has a therapeutic effect on the ankles, knees and thighs.

The process of resting the mind and temporarily stopping its usual frantic activity is known in the study of Yoga as "meditation." The Yogis have used the LOTUS positions for thousands of years for the practice of meditation. When you grow accustomed to one of the LOTUS postures, you will experience the profound and complete relaxation which it provides, especially if you practice in a quiet place without distractions, close your eyes and attempt to stop your thoughts for a number of minutes. The practice of meditation is a most effective manner of overcoming nervousness, fear and anxiety.

Points To Remember When Practicing the Lotus Postures

1. Be patient. Some areas of the feet, ankles, legs and knees will feel uncomfortable in the beginning. This indicates they have grown weak, stiff and tense. If you will simply accommodate your legs, ankles and feet as best you can, you will find that you progress quickly.

2. Sit erectly at all times. Do not allow yourself to slump.

3. When your legs grow tired, stretch them straight out, massage your knees gently with your hands and then reverse the legs and resume the posture.

4. As your legs gain in flexibility, attempt to change gradually from the cross-legged posture to the HALF-LOTUS or from the HALF-LOTUS to the FULL-LOTUS. Hold the FULL-LOTUS for only a few seconds in the beginning.

5. For the practice of *meditation,* close your eyes and attempt to stop your thoughts for several minutes. Stopping the thoughts is not easy. It requires daily practice.

The plan of practice for the 6 techniques of this first week is given below. Practice these techniques at least once each day. Practice twice each day whenever possible.

If the number of seconds given to hold a posture seems too difficult for you, you may modify the plan in accordance with your ability.

Practice very easily whenever you are stiff.*

If you are not certain of how to do any of the movements of a particular technique, go back and read the instructions of that technique again. It is very important that you learn the technique correctly.

No.	Name	Times	Hold
1	PRELIMINARY LEG PULL	3	10 sec.
2	KNEE AND THIGH STRETCH	3	15 sec.* *
3	BACKWARD BEND	2 feet	10 sec.
		1 toes	10 sec.
4	TOE TWIST	2 both sides	10 sec.
5	ARM AND LEG STRETCH	2 both sides	10 sec.* *
6	LOTUS POSTURES	whenever possible; alternate the legs	as long as comfortable

* Progress in Yoga is such that the body is continually changing as it gradually stretches and becomes flexible and strong. Therefore you may experience some slight discomfort from time to time. This is natural and practically universal with everyone who practices physical Yoga. If you simply relax and practice easily during these periods you will find that they do not last long.

** This is the final duration for this technique. No additional time will be added.

SECOND WEEK

On the first and second days of this Second Week carefully learn the 3 techniques listed below. Continue to practice the 6 techniques you have already learned according to page 58.

       7.   CHEST EXPANSION

       8.   COBRA

       9.   NECK MOVEMENTS

On the third day of this week turn to page 73 and begin your practice according to the 'Practice Plan' for this Second Week.

YOUTH
through *NATURAL DEVELOPMENT*

● Technique No. 7—CHEST EXPANSION

What the Chest Expansion Posture Does for You

1. Develops the chest, bust and seldom-exercised muscles of the shoulders.

2. Expands the lungs and stimulates the lung cells.

3. Provides a quick relief of tension throughout the trunk.

4. Aids in a general improvement of the posture.

How To Do the Chest Expansion

1. Stand easily with your arms at your sides.

2. Bend your elbows and raise your arms *slowly* so that the back of your hands touch your chest.

3. Now straighten out your arms at chest level and bring them back slowly until you can clasp your hands behind your back. Straighten out your clasped hands and arms as far as you can without discomfort. Remain standing erectly; *do not bend forward.*

4. Keeping your hands clasped and your arms held high, *slowly and easily* bend *backward* from the waist. Drop the head backward a few inches and look upward. Go only as far backward as you can without strain and hold this position for 5 seconds. (Fig. 15)

5. Now *slowly* bend forward at the waist. Bring your clasped hands and arms up stiffly over your back as you

bend forward. Keep your knees straight and allow your neck muscles to relax as though you would touch your forehead to your knees. Remain in your extreme forward position without motion for 10 seconds.   (Fig. 16)

6. *Slowly* straighten to the upright position. When you are standing erectly once again, unclasp your hands and stand easily with your arms at your sides. Rest several moments without becoming restless and repeat as advised.

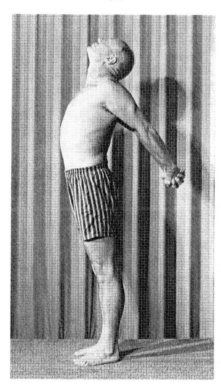

Fig. 15

Fig. 16

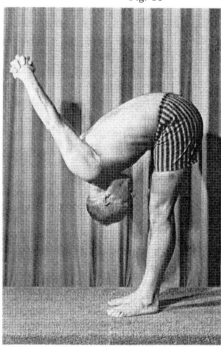

How To Practice the Chest Expansion

Time to hold the extreme
positions: backward: 5 seconds
                                forward: 10 seconds
Number of times: 2
Time of the day: AM and/or PM

Important Things To Know About the Chest Expansion

As with the ARM AND LEG STRETCH, this is another excellent technique which you may do whenever you feel the discomfort of tension. The CHEST EXPANSION posture is therefore excellent for people whose work requires them to spend long periods of time sitting. The backward and forward bends of this technique reach many key tension points in the body and will remove tightness and the feeling of being cramped. The movement of the arms also develops seldom-exercised muscles in the arms and shoulders. In the forward bend, the blood is allowed to flow into the head, helping to revitalize the brain. This technique is excellent for stimulating the lung cells and improving the posture. A natural development of the chest area will occur. Take advantage of the wonderful stimulating effects of this exercise by doing it several times each day, especially during a "break" in working hours.

Points To Remember When Practicing the Chest Expansion

1. Move your arms slowly and gracefully at all times and in step 3 keep them *high* as you bring them back.

2. During step 3 remain standing upright. Do not allow your trunk to bend forward.

3. Once your hands are clasped, keep your arms as high as possible throughout the remainder of the exercise.

4. In the backward bend of step 4 be very cautious and do not strain. Hold only for 5 seconds as instructed. Breathe normally.

5. In the forward bend remember to move your arms up over your back as far as possible and hold them there during the 10-second count.

6. Remember to straighten up *very slowly* and do not unclasp your hands until you are once again in the upright position.

YOUTH
for the *BACK*

● Technique No. 8—COBRA

What the Cobra Does for You

1. Stimulates and relaxes the vertebrae from the neck to the base of the spine.

2. Provides a methodical relief of tension and stiffness throughout the back. (This posture is excellent for relaxing the body before retiring.)

3. Develops the chest and bust and strengthens the muscles of the back and buttocks.

4. Aids in a general improvement of the posture.

How To Do the Cobra

1. Lie on your abdomen with your face resting on your cheek and your arms at your sides. Close your eyes and allow your body to go completely limp.

2. Turn your head so that your forehead rests on the floor.

3. Use only your neck muscles to *slowly* raise your head upward and backward as far as it will go.

4. Keep your head back and *slowly* raise your trunk from the floor as far as you can, using only your back muscles to aid you. (Fig. 17)

5. When you have raised your trunk to its limit, bring your hands in from your sides and place them beneath your upper chest, the fingers of both hands pointing toward one another. (See Fig. 18 for this hand position.)

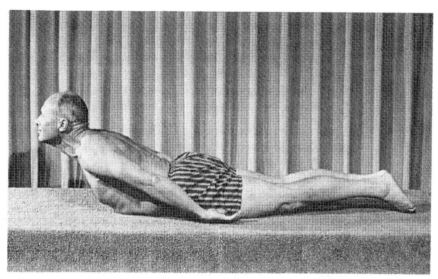

Fig. 17

Fig. 18

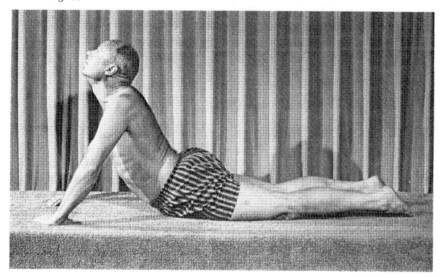

6. Now using your hands for support, *slowly* raise your trunk as far from the floor as possible. Your spine must be *continually curved* during this raising and your head must be held back. Try to feel each vertebra stretch during this movement. *Stop at whatever point this movement becomes a strain.*

7. The ultimate position will eventually be reached when your abdomen is raised from the floor and your body is resting on the groin. (Fig. 18) Wherever you stop this movement, hold your position *motionless* for the advised number of seconds.

8. At the completion of the count, *slowly* lower your trunk making sure it is continually curved as you come down. Your head moves slowly forward.

9. When you can support your trunk without the aid of your hands, return them to your sides as in Fig. 17.

10. Continue to lower your trunk and head. When your forehead touches the floor, pause for a moment and then turn your cheek to rest on the floor as you began this exercise. Relax for approximately one minute and then proceed to the NECK MOVEMENTS.

How To Practice the Cobra

Time to hold the extreme position:	begin with 10 seconds; add the seconds as advised in future weeks until 20 seconds are reached.
Number of times:	3; each cobra is followed by the Neck Movement
Time of the day:	PM

Important Things To Know About the Cobra

Careful practice of the COBRA will return the youthful "spring" and vitality throughout your back and spine. I advise my students to practice the COBRA when they return home from work or from any tiring activity which leaves them tense and fatigued. The manner in which the COBRA begins with the neck area and methodically works downward to the base of the spine, simultaneously stimulates and relaxes each of the vertebrae. This type of relaxation proves extremely refreshing and enables you to regain vitality. It is a good technique to do before retiring if you are troubled with insomnia. If you practice as advised you will be able to raise your trunk a little further each day. You need do the COBRA only a few times properly to experience its immediate effects.

Points To Remember When Practicing the Cobra

1. Move in absolute *slow-motion.*

2. Keep your spine continually *curved* as you raise and lower your trunk.

3. Your head should bend backward while raising your trunk.

4. Make certain that you have the correct position of your hands by consulting Fig. 18.

5. Raise your trunk only as far as you can comfortably. Do not strain. The vertebrae will "give" gradually.

6. Carefully count the correct number of seconds in the extreme position. Always be exact about your count in each technique.

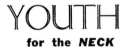

for the *NECK*

● **Technique No. 9—NECK MOVEMENTS**

What the Neck Movements Do for You

1. Remove stiffness and tension in the neck.

2. Strengthen the muscles of the neck.

How To Do the Neck Movements

The NECK MOVEMENTS will always follow the COBRA

1. After you have finished the COBRA and rested, prop yourself up on your elbows as you see in Fig. 19. Place your hands and fingers securely on the *back* of your head. Gently push down until your chin rests on the top of your chest or as close to it as possible. Hold this position for the prescribed 20 seconds. (Fig. 19)

2. *Slowly* raise your head. With hardly any movement of your hands, place your chin in your left palm and place your right hand securely on the back of your head. *Slowly* turn your head as far to the left as is possible without strain and hold this position without movement for the prescribed 20 seconds. (Fig. 20)

3. *Slowly* turn your head so that you can now rest your chin in your right palm and place your left hand securely on the back of your head. *Slowly* turn your head as far to the right as is possible without strain and hold this position for the prescribed 20 seconds.

4. Slowly return your arms to your sides; lie down once again and rest your cheek on the floor.

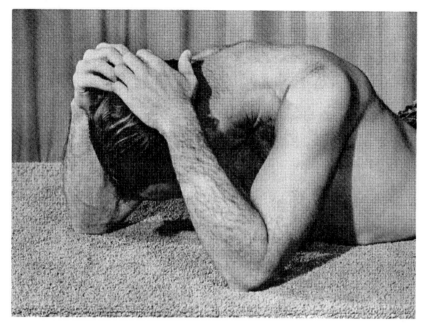

Fig. 19

Fig. 20

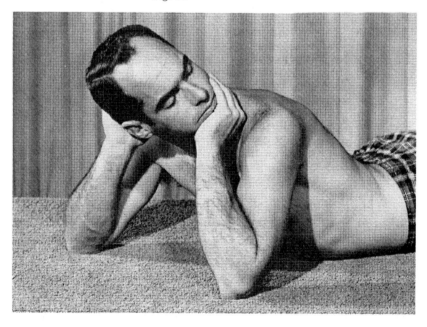

How To Practice the Neck Movements

Time to hold the extreme
positions: 20 seconds each

Number of times each   3; one series following each
movement: COBRA.

Time of the day: PM

Important Things To Know About the Neck Movements

A very great tension point, the neck is often stiff and cramped. You have probably seen people going through various gyrations of the neck, rolling it to and fro in an attempt to loosen some of the tightness. But quick movements will never truly remove tension. If you are troubled with a stiff and tense neck, you will find that these methodical neck movements will provide wonderful relief.

Points To Remember When Practicing the Neck Movements

1. Make sure that your hands grip your head firmly in all movements.

2. Keep your arms close together; your elbows remain on the floor at all times.

3. Do not make any quick or sudden movements in turning your head. Do not strain.

4. Hold your head in the extreme positions without motion. Close your eyes and count the seconds silently.

The 9 techniques you have now learned are grouped below under 'A' and 'B'. There are 2 methods of practicing these groups. Choose that method which you find most suitable.

Method 1—Practice *twice* each day. Do group A in the AM (before breakfast, mid-morning, noontime). Do group B in the PM (afternoon, before dinner, later at night).

Method 2—Practice *once* each day. Do group A on one day and group B the next day. Go back to group A on the third day and continue to alternate during the remainder of the week. If you miss a day of practice, resume on the following day where you left off. For example, if you do group A on Tuesday and are unable to practice on Wednesday, resume your practice on Thursday with group B. Keep a record of your practice days on a separate sheet of paper so that you always know the correct group to do.

If the number of seconds given to hold a posture seems too difficult for you, you may modify the plan in accordance with your ability.

Practice very easily whenever you are stiff.

If you are not certain of how to do any of the movements of a particular technique, go back and read the instructions of that technique again. It is very important that you learn the techniques correctly.

Group A

No.	Name	Times	Hold
1	PRELIMINARY LEG PULL	3	10 sec
2	KNEE AND THIGH STRETCH	3	15 sec*
3	BACKWARD BEND	2 feet 1 toes	10 sec 10 sec
4	TOE TWIST	2 both sides	10 sec
5	ARM AND LEG STRETCH	2 both sides	10 sec*
6	LOTUS POSTURES	whenever possible; alternate the legs	as long as comfortable

Group B

No.	Name	Times	Hold
7	CHEST EXPANSION	2	backward: 5 sec* forward: 10 sec*
8	COBRA	3	10 sec
9	NECK MOVEMENTS	3; (one series after each COBRA)	20 seconds each movement*

---

*This is the final duration for this technique. No additional time will be added.

THIRD WEEK

On the first and second days of this Third Week carefully learn the 3 techniques listed below. Continue to practice the 9 techniques you have already learned according to page 73.

      10.   COMPLETE BREATH
      11.   SHOULDER STAND
      12.   EYE EXERCISES

On the third day of this week turn to page 91 and begin your practice according to the 'Practice Plan' for this Third Week.

REVITALIZATION
through *COMPLETE BREATHING*

● **Technique No. 10—COMPLETE BREATH**

What the Complete Breath Does for You

1. Helps to purify and improve the quality of the blood.

2. Increases resistance to colds and other respiratory diseases.

3. Expands the chest cavity, develops the diaphragm and imparts a general improvement in health and appearance.

4. Strengthens the nervous system and lends alertness and clarity to the mind by supplying an increased amount of life-force *(prana)*.

How To Do the Complete Breath

Our objective in this technique is to fill the lungs with air. In order to do this it is necessary to make several movements of the body during the breathing.

1. Sit in a cross-legged posture. Breathe normally. First we will learn only the physical movements. The first of these movements is to use your abdominal muscles to push your abdomen out as far as possible. (Fig. 21) This movement will enable the air to be taken into the lower lungs during breathing.

2. Practice pulling in with the abdomen and pushing out first in the lower chest and then the upper chest areas. (Fig. 22) Finally, raise your shoulders, keeping your hands on your knees. (Fig. 23)

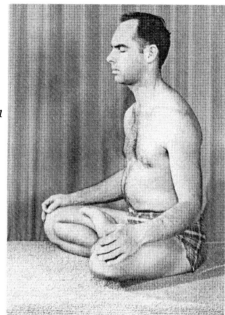

Fig. 21

Fig. 22

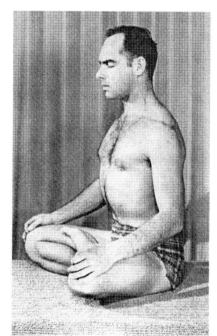

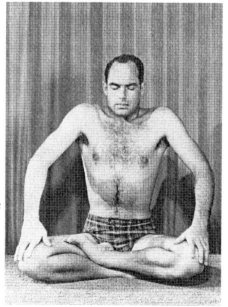

Fig. 23

3. Slowly lower your shoulders and relax your chest and abdomen.

4. Practice to make step 1 flow easily into step 2.

5. Next, practice only the breathing. First exhale completely through your nose so that there is no air in your lungs. Now inhale slowly, so slowly that it will take you 15 seconds to complete your inhalation. Count these seconds silently. (It may take a few attempts to slow down your breathing sufficiently so that you can accomplish your inhalation within 15 seconds.)

6. Retain the air in your lungs for 10 seconds. Count the seconds carefully.

7. Exhale through your nose during a count of 15 seconds.

8. Practice steps 5, 6 and 7 until the count of 15-10-15 is mastered.

9. Now combine the physical movements of steps 1, 2 and 3 with the breathing of steps 5, 6 and 7: push out with the abdomen as you inhale during the first 5 seconds. Next pull in with your abdomen and push out in the chest areas during the second group of 5 seconds. Finally, raise your shoulders during the last 5 seconds. Retain the air for 10 seconds. Exhale slowly through your nose and return to the normal position during a count of 15 seconds.

10. When the lungs are empty, repeat as advised.

How To Practice the Complete Breath

Time for execution of the
movements:

inhale—5 seconds for the
abdominal area;
5 seconds for the
chest areas;
5 seconds to lift the
shoulders;
retain—10 seconds;
exhale—15 seconds.

Number of times: 5 to 10 (as time permits)

Time of the day:
(1) whenever possible during the day;
(2) as advised in the "Practice Plans."

Important Things To Know About the Complete Breath

The way in which you breathe directly affects your physical
and mental well-being and determines to a great extent the
length and quality of your life. Most people have the habit
of shallow breathing, using only the high breathing area.
The COMPLETE BREATH makes full use of the lungs and
consequently must improve the quality of your blood, complexion, appearance, general health and aids in alertness
and clarity of mind. You should take a few COMPLETE
BREATHS whenever you can during the day. If you do not
make the exaggerated motions of raising your shoulders as
described in step 2, you will find it is possible to take the
COMPLETE BREATH without drawing attention to yourself. Consequently, it can be done almost anywhere and at
any time when you wish to revitalize your body and clear
your mind.

Points To Remember When Practicing the Complete Breath

1. Learn to make the 3 physical movements of the inhalation flow smoothly into one another.

2. The inhalation is continuous; do not stop the inhalation until the lungs have been completely filled during the 15 second count.

3. Inhale and exhale in a very controlled manner so that you cannot hear the air going in or coming out of the nostrils. (This control will aid you in inhaling as slowly as necessary.)

4. All breathing is done through the nose.

5. Make sure that the air is completely exhaled and your lungs empty before you begin your next inhalation. Contracting your abdomen at the end of the exhalation will force all air from the lower lungs and help make the exhalation complete.

6. Close your eyes throughout the exercise and count all movements carefully.

YOUTH

through *CONTROLLED WEIGHT AND RELAXATION OF STRAINED AREAS*

● Technique No. 11—SHOULDER STAND

What the Shoulder Stand Does for You

1. Aids in the control of weight through its reaction on the thyroid gland.

2. Helps to improve the blood circulation.

3. Allows many vital organs and glands to revert to their proper position.

4. Relaxes the legs and other strained areas through a relief of pressure.

How To Do the Shoulder Stand

1. Lie flat on your back with your arms at your sides. Allow your body to go limp; close your eyes; breathe normally.

2. Turn your palms downward so that they press against the floor. Bring your legs together and tense your leg and abdominal muscles.

3. Slowly raise your legs up into the air until they are at a right angle with the floor. (Performing this movement slowly will help to strengthen and firm the thighs and abdomen.)

4. Keep your knees stiff; press down hard on the floor with your palms; swing your legs easily back over your head. This movement should enable you to raise the lower part

of your back from the floor so that you can support your lumbar region with your hands. (Fig. 24)

5. *Slowly and carefully* attempt to straighten yourself as far as you can into a vertical position. Stop wherever the posture becomes a strain. The ultimate position will be seen in Fig. 25. Hold your extreme position for the prescribed time. You need not hold your body rigid or tense in the vertical position. You should attempt to relax as much as possible.

6. To return your body to the floor, first bend your legs at the knees and bring your knees as close as you can down toward your forehead. Next, place your hands on the floor and support yourself. (Fig. 26) Now roll forward and arch your neck so that you can keep the back of your head and your back on the floor.

7. When your lower back is resting on the floor, extend your legs straight out into the air and slowly lower them to the floor.

8. Allow your body to go completely limp and rest for at least one minute.

Fig. 24

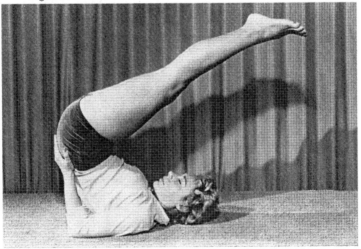

Fig. 25

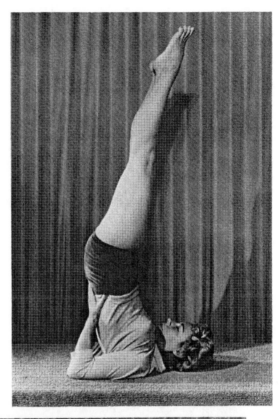

Fig. 26

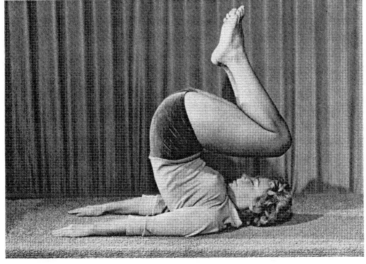

How To Practice the Shoulder Stand

Time to hold the extreme
position:

begin with 1 minute; add the seconds as advised in future weeks until 3 minutes are reached. You can eventually hold the Shoulder Stand for 5 minutes and longer if you experience no strain.

Number of times: 1

Time of the day: AM and/or PM

Important Things To Know About the Shoulder Stand

Inverting the body for relaxation and to promote good blood circulation is one of the finest Yoga concepts. The SHOULDER STAND and the HEAD STAND are used for this purpose. One of these should be done every day. Gravity is continually at work upon your body exerting its pull on many vital organs and glands and causing the blood to flow predominately downward. The SHOULDER STAND inverts the body and allows the blood to flow freely through those areas in which circulation may be poor. In this inverted position many organs and glands relax. The SHOULDER STAND also has a positive effect upon the thyroid gland which acts as an aid to weight control.

If you have difficulty in raising your lower back from the floor as described in step 4, try swinging your legs quickly backward to give yourself some momentum. You can always use the wall for aid. Simply "walk" up the wall as far as you can comfortably and hold whatever angle you can attain for the prescribed time. In the beginning any angle of inversion is beneficial. Little by little you will gain sufficient strength to do the SHOULDER STAND with your own power. You will find that this posture has a wonderful *revitalizing* effect as well.

Points To Remember When Practicing the Shoulder Stand

1. Always raise your leg slowly and stiffly from the floor; this movement helps tone the abdominal muscles.

2. Attempt gradually to invert your body as straight as possible. This final position is shown in Fig. 25 where the chin is touching the chest.

3. Do not fidget or move excessively while in the SHOUL-DER STAND; you need not hold your body absolutely rigid or tense. Relax. Also keep your mind on your breathing; inhale and exhale very slowly.

4. Close your eyes but keep a watch or a clock nearby so that you may glance at it once or twice for time elapsed. Add the seconds to this posture exactly as advised each week.

5. Make every attempt to come out of the SHOULDER STAND exactly as described in the instructions in steps 6, 7, and 8. These movements should be performed with control, grace and balance. Remember to arch your neck backward so that your head can remain on the floor as you roll forward in step 6.

6. Always rest in the reclining position for at least 1 minute.

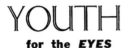

for the *EYES*

● Technique No. 12—EYE EXERCISES

What the Eye Exercises Do for You

1. Have a positive effect upon the optic nerves and muscles.

2. Aid in relieving tension and fatigue of the eyes often responsible for headaches.

How To Do the Eye Exercises

1. Imagine that you are facing the center of a **giant** clock. In order to see twelve o'clock you would have to move your eyes (without moving your head) to the position of Fig. 27.

2. In order to see one o'clock you would have to move your eyes slightly to the upper *right*-hand corner; to see two o'clock you would move your eyes a little farther to the right; to see three o'clock you would move to the position of Fig. 28, and so forth around the clock. On each number you must *rest your eyes for a fraction of a second.*
Perform this clockwise movement 10 times, resting for a moment on each of the 12 numbers.

3. When 10 clockwise movements are completed, close your eyes and rest for several seconds. Then open your eyes and do the identical movements in a counter-clockwise fashion 10 times. In this movement you begin at twelve o'clock as before, but move the eyes to your *left* so that you see eleven o'clock, then ten o'clock, etc.

4. When 10 counter-clockwise movements are completed, close your eyes and rest for several moments.

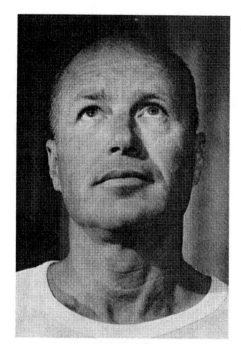

Fig. 27

Fig. 28

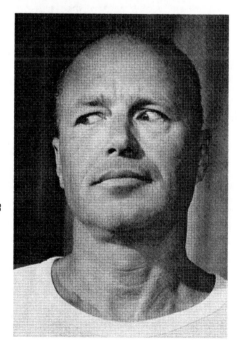

How To Practice the Eye Exercises

Time to hold the extreme positions:	a fraction-of-a-second stop on each of the 12 numbers.
Number of times:	10 clockwise movements; 10 counter-clockwise movements.
Time of the day:	PM

Important Things To Know About the Eye Exercises

The optic nerves and muscles are usually neglected in ordinary exercising. Since with our Yoga techniques, we are reconditioning every part of the body, we should certainly make some conscious effort to exercise the eye muscles a few times each week. Moving the eyes to the extreme areas of the socket as described will provide this exercise. You will also find that fatigue of the eyes is often relieved through these movements.

Points To Remember When Practicing the Eye Exercises

1. Make sure that your eyes are being moved to the extreme areas of the socket.

2. Pause for a fraction of a second on each number.

3. Close your eyes for several moments when the clockwise group is complete. Then open your eyes and perform the counter-clockwise group. Rest your eyes for several minutes after the exercise is completed.

The 12 techniques you have now learned are grouped below under 'A' and 'B.' From this point on, the order in which you are learning the techniques is not necessarily the order in which they will be practiced.

There are 2 methods of practicing these groups. Choose that method which you find most suitable.

> *Method 1*—Practice *twice* each day. Do group A in the AM (before breakfast, mid-morning, noontime). Do group B in the PM (afternoon, before dinner, later at night).

> *Method 2*—Practice *once* each day. Do group A on one day and group B the next day. Go back to group A on the third day and continue to alternate during the remainder of the week. If you miss a day of practice, resume on the following day where you left off. For example, if you do group A on Tuesday and are unable to practice on Wednesday, resume your practice on Thursday with group B. Keep a record of your practice days on a separate sheet of paper so that you always know the correct group to do.

If the number of seconds given to hold a posture seems too difficult for you, you may modify the plan in accordance with your ability.

Practice very easily whenever you are stiff.

If you are not certain of how to do any of the movements of a particular technique, go back and read the instructions of that technique again. It is very important that you learn the techniques correctly.

Group A

No.	Name	Times	Hold
1	PRELIMINARY LEG PULL	3	20 sec°
2	KNEE AND THIGH	3	15 sec°
3	BACKWARD BEND	2 feet 1 toes	15 sec 15 sec
4	TOE TWIST	2 both sides	10 sec
5	ARM AND LEG STRETCH	2 both sides	10 sec°
7	CHEST EXPANSION	2	backward: 5 sec° forward: 10 sec°
10	COMPLETE BREATH (seated in one of the Lotus postures)	5 - 10	inhale: 15 sec° retain: 10 sec° exhale: 15 sec°

Group B

8	COBRA	3	10 sec
9	NECK MOVEMENTS	3; (one series after each COBRA)	20 sec each movement°
11	SHOULDER STAND	1	1 minute
12	EYE EXERCISES (seated in one of the Lotus postures)	10 clockwise; 10 counter-clockwise	a fraction-of-a-sec-hold on each of the 12 num-bers°
10	COMPLETE BREATH (seated in one of the Lotus postures)	5 - 10	as in Group A

° This is the final duration for this technique. No additional time will be added.

Notes: Sit in one of the Lotus postures whenever you can during the day. Do the COMPLETE BREATH, ARM AND LEG STRETCH and CHEST EXPANSION at any time of the day when you desire relief from fatigue and tension.

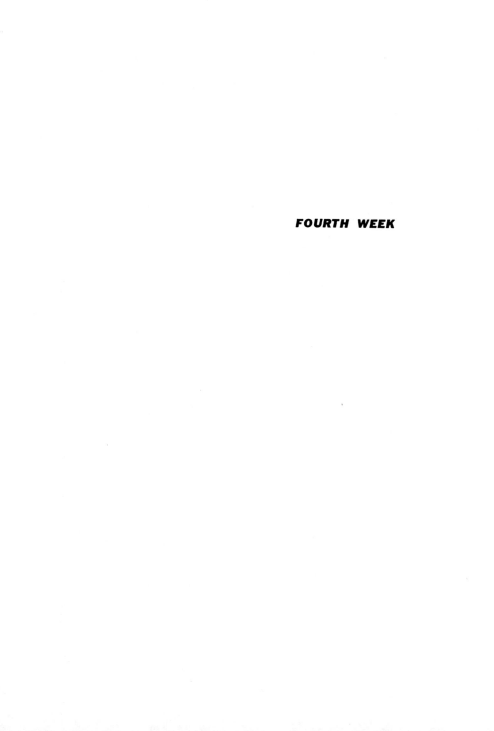

FOURTH WEEK

On the first and second days of this Fourth Week carefully learn the 2 techniques listed below. Continue to practice the 12 techniques you have already learned according to page 91.

13. ABDOMINAL LIFT
14. ALTERNATE NOSTRIL BREATHING

On the third day of this week turn to page 106 and begin your practice according to the 'Practice Plan' for this Fourth Week.

YOUTH

through *STIMULATION OF INTERNAL ORGANS AND GLANDS*

● Technique No. 13—ABDOMINAL LIFT

What the Abdominal Lift Does for You

1. Has a positive reaction on the stomach, colon, intestines, liver, kidneys, gall bladder, pancreas and reproductive organs and glands.

2. Helps to promote the peristaltic action relieving and preventing constipation.

3. Reduces flabbiness in the waist and maintains the resilience of the abdominal muscles thus helping to prevent the abdomen from dropping.

How To Do the Abdominal Lift

1. Study Figs. 29 and 30. It is important to realize that the lifting of the abdomen can be accomplished successfully only if all air is first exhaled from the lungs and no air is allowed to enter while the abdominal movements are being performed.

2. Place your body in the position of Fig. 30. Notice that the hands are placed high on the thighs with the fingers of both hands pointing inward. The knees are bent and the body is in a slight squatting position.

3. Exhale all air from your lungs and hold it out as you attempt to lift the abdomen as depicted in Fig. 29. Perhaps the best way of describing this movement

is to say that it is a "sucking" of the abdomen inward and upward. It is as though you were trying to breathe very deeply beginning from the abdominal area. No air actually enters your lungs but the abdominal area goes through the motions of this deep breath, during which it is sucked inward and upward.

4. Hold the lift for a few moments and then attempt to "snap" the abdomen out by using the abdominal muscles.

5. Repeat this movement without allowing any air to enter your lungs. Do 3 of these lifts with each exhalation. Five movements will become easy with a little practice.

6. When the movements are completed stand upright and breathe easily for a few moments. Then go back into the squatting position and repeat.

Fig. 29

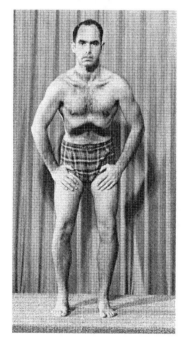

Fig. 30

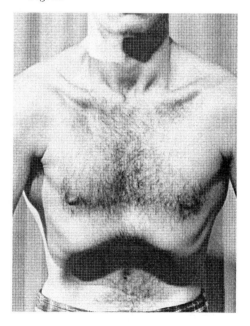

How To Practice the Abdominal Lift

Time to hold the lift:	approximately 3 seconds
Number of times:	begin with 3 movements during each exhalation and perform this 5 times so that you do 15 movements in all. Add 1 movement each week until you reach 5 movements during each exhalation. Perform these 5 movements 5 times so that you do 25 movements in all. Although 25 is an adequate number you may eventually do as many as 50 movements if desired.
Time of the day:	AM and/or PM — always with an empty stomach. Before breakfast is actually the best time.

Important Things To Know About the Abdominal Lift

The ABDOMINAL LIFT is the very finest natural movement you can perform to stimulate and promote the correct functioning of the vital visceral organs and glands. Success in this exercise is simply a matter of practice and you must not be discouraged if you are not able to perform the "lift" completely during the first few days. The technique may seem peculiar at first until you catch on to the knack of doing the movements *while the breath is exhaled.* All of the breath must be exhaled and held out in order to form a vacuum or you will not be able to lift sufficiently.

However, if in the beginning you are able only to *contract* your abdomen slightly you are on the road to success and you will already find yourself benefiting from this movement. I cannot speak too highly of the therapeutic value of this technique.

Points To Remember When Practicing the Abdominal Lift

1. Remember that the eventual goal is not only to *contract* the abdomen; it is both to contract and *raise* it.

2. The abdomen is not allowed simply to "fall" back to its normal position. It is "shot" or "snapped" out in a forceful movement by the abdominal muscles.

3. These movements are done forcefully and rhythmically. Keep a steady rhythm. In the very beginning you may wish to do only 1 movement to each exhalation and work up gradually to 2 and 3 movements. It is the steady rhythm which is important, not the speed.

4. Note carefully the position of the body, hands, legs, etc., in Fig. 29. Do not allow yourself to lean over farther than you see in the illustration.

5. When you stand up to rest after each group, try not to fidget or grow restless. Simply stand quietly for a few moments until you are rested and then repeat.

YOUTH
through *RELIEF FROM NERVOUSNESS, ANXIETY, INSOMNIA*

● Technique No. 14—ALTERNATE NOSTRIL
                                BREATHING

What Alternate Nostril Breathing Does for You

1. Imparts an immediate sensation of tranquility and calmness to the entire body and mind.

2. Helps to overcome nervousness, anxiety and insomnia.

3. Restores equilibrium in cases of emotional upsets.

4. Greatly aids in relieving headaches.

How To Do Alternate Nostril Breathing

1. Look at Fig. 31 and note the position of the hands and fingers. Assume this position with your right hand. Keep your hand relaxed.

2. Close your right nostril by pressing it with your right thumb and exhale all of the air in your lungs through your left nostril.

3. Inhale slowly through your left nostril and attempt to fill your lungs in a rhythmic count of 8 beats.

4. Press your left nostril closed with your ring finger so that both nostrils are now closed. Retain the air in your lungs for a rhythmic count of 8 beats. (Fig. 32) Count the seconds silently.

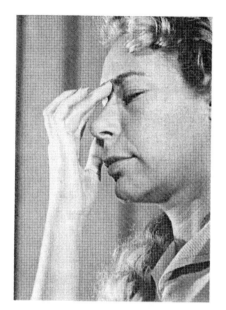

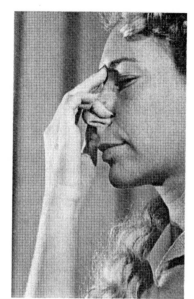

Fig. 31   Fig. 32

5. Open your right nostril by gently releasing your thumb and attempt to exhale completely through your right nostril during a rhythmic count of 8 beats. Count the seconds silently and rhythmically.

6. Without pause, begin the next group of 8 beats and without moving your fingers begin to inhale fully, this time through your *right* nostril. (This is the same nostril through which you just finished exhaling.)

7. Press the right nostril closed with your thumb so that both nostrils are now closed. Retain the air in your lungs during the next rhythmic count of 8 beats. Count silently and rhythmically.

8. Open your left nostril by gently releasing your ring finger and exhale through your left nostril during the next rhythmic count of 8 beats. When you finish this group you will be back to the starting position. This completes *one round* of this technique.

9. Without pause, begin the next round by proceeding as in step 3.

10. Do the prescribed number of rounds; count silently and rhythmically. When you have finished, lower your hand; keep your eyes closed; relax.

How To Practice Alternate Nostril Breathing

Time for the 3 parts:	inhalation: count of 8
	retention: count of 8
	exhalation: count of 8
Number of times:	5 rounds. Look back to your instructions to make sure you understand the word "round."
Time of the day:	whenever needed for tranquility and calmness.

Important Things To Know About Alternate Nostril Breathing

Here is a truly remarkable technique for quieting, calming and relieving tension and negative feelings. It may be somewhat of a mystery to you as to how this method of breathing is able so to relax the body and mind, but you have only to follow the instructions to realize its benefits. I advise my students to practice this form of breathing as soon as possible after an upsetting experience. It quickly restores equilibrium and is wonderful for dispelling fear and anxiety. ALTERNATE NOSTRIL BREATHING has also helped many people to overcome insomnia and other forms of nervousness as well as relieve headaches and nasal congestion. This technique will become one of your most powerful natural weapons for coping with physical and mental tensions of the everyday world.

**Points To Remember When Practicing
Alternate Nostril Breathing**

1. Always practice this technique privately in the most quiet surroundings possible.

2. Remember to sit erectly and count the groups of 8 carefully to yourself. A steady rhythm in this technique is most important.

3. Control the breath as much as possible. Try not to let it rush in or out of the nostrils.

4. Keep your right hand relaxed.

5. It is best to sit in the Lotus, or cross-legged posture when practicing this breathing, but if this position becomes too tiring you may assume any other comfortable position. It can be done sitting in a chair and even lying down.

The 14 techniques you have now learned are grouped below under 'A' and 'B.'

There are 2 methods of practicing these groups. Choose that method which you find most suitable.

> *Method 1*—Practice *twice* each day. Do group A in the AM (before breakfast, mid-morning, noontime). Do group B in the PM (afternoon, before dinner, later at night).
>
> *Method 2*—Practice *once* each day. Do group A on one day and group B the next day. Go back to group A on the third day and continue to alternate during the remainder of the week. If you miss a day of practice, resume on the following day where you left off. For example, if you do group A on Tuesday and are unable to practice on Wednesday, resume your practice on Thursday with group B. Keep a record of your practice days on a separate sheet of paper so that you always know the correct group to do.

If the number of seconds given to hold a posture seems too difficult for you, you may modify the plan in accordance with your ability.

Practice very easily whenever you are stiff.

If you are not certain of how to do any of the movements of a particular technique, go back and read the instructions of that technique again. It is very important that you learn the techniques correctly.

Group A

No.	Name	Times	Hold
1	PRELIMINARY LEG PULL	3	20 sec°
2	KNEE AND THIGH STRETCH	3	15 sec°
3	BACKWARD BEND	2 feet 1 toes	15 sec 15 sec
4	TOE TWIST	2 both sides	10 sec
5	ARM AND LEG STRETCH	2 both sides	10 sec°
7	CHEST EXPANSION	2	backward: 5 sec° forward: 10 sec°
13	ABDOMINAL LIFT	15 (5x3)	approx. 3 seconds each lift°
10	COMPLETE BREATH (seated in one of the Lotus postures)	5 - 10	inhale: 15 sec° retain: 10 sec° exhale: 15 sec°

Group B

No.	Name	Times	Hold
8	**COBRA**	3	15 seconds
9	**NECK MOVEMENTS**	3; (one series after each COBRA)	20 seconds each movement°
11	**SHOULDER STAND**	1	1½ minutes
12	**EYE EXERCISES** (seated in one of the Lotus postures)	10 clockwise; 10 counter-clockwise	a fraction-of-a-second hold on each of the 12 numbers°
14	**ALTERNATE NOS-TRIL BREATHING** (seated in one of the Lotus postures)	5 rounds	inhale: count of 8° retain: count of 8° exhale: count of 8°

° This is the final duration for this technique. No additional time will be added.

Notes: Sit in one of the Lotus postures whenever you can during the day. Do the COMPLETE BREATH, ARM AND LEG STRETCH, CHEST EXPANSION and ALTERNATE NOSTRIL BREATH-ING at any time of the day when you desire relief from fatigue, tension, anxiety.

FIFTH WEEK

On the first and second days of this Fifth Week carefully learn the 2 techniques listed below. Continue to practice the 14 techniques you have already learned according to page 106.

      15.   LOCUST
      16.   BOW

On the third day of this week turn to page 120 and begin your practice according to the 'Practice Plan' for this Fifth Week.

YOUTH

through *STRENGTHENING NEGLECTED MUSCLES IN THE ABDOMEN, LEGS AND ARMS*

● Technique No. 15—LOCUST

What the Locust Does for You

1. Develops and strengthens the abdomen, legs, buttocks and arms.

2. Improves the blood circulation.

3. Helps to reduce weight in the thighs and hips and makes the skin in these areas taut and firm.

4. Stimulates the thyroid, liver, intestines, kidneys and reproductive organs and glands.

How To Do the Locust

The LOCUST always follows the COBRA and the NECK MOVEMENTS.

1. When you have finished the NECK MOVEMENTS and are once again lying on your abdomen with your cheek resting on the floor and your arms at your sides, you are ready to perform the LOCUST.

2. Turn your head and rest your *chin* on the floor. (In the COBRA it was the forehead which rested on the floor to begin the posture.)

3. Make fists with both hands and place them thumbs down near your sides. See the illustrations for the position of the fists.

4. Inhale so that your lungs are about half full and your chest is slightly expanded. Retain the air in your lungs.

5. Holding the air, push down with your fists and lift your legs as far from the floor as you can with your knees held as straight as possible. Throw the weight of your legs up toward your chin and balance yourself with your chin and both fists. Hold for the prescribed count. Fig. 33 represents an elementary stage of this posture and Fig. 34 is a more advanced position which comes with practice.

6. *Slowly* return your legs to the floor and exhale through your nose. Control this movement and do not allow the air to rush out.

7. Rest your cheek on the floor and relax.

Fig. 33

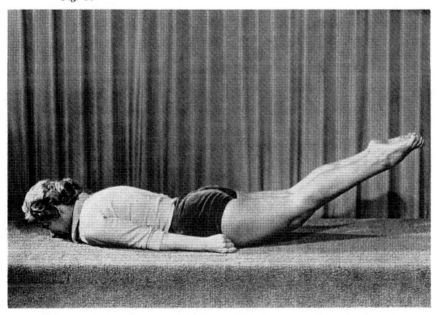

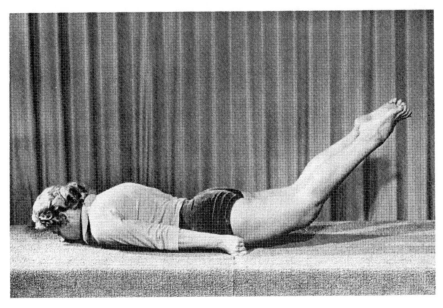

Fig. 34

How To Practice the Locust

Time to hold the extreme position:	begin with 5 seconds; add the seconds as advised in future weeks until 10 seconds are reached.
Number of times:	3; once following each set of the COBRA and NECK MOVEMENTS
Time of the day:	PM

Important Things To Know About the Locust

This is a wonderful developing technique which will strengthen and give you control of very important muscles that you have almost certainly neglected through the years. In looking at the photographs you can see the muscles in the abdomen, legs and arms which are used in this posture.

It is simply the repeated attempts which will gradually develop these weak areas. This movement will lend firmness and strength and help to streamline your body without placing undue strain on the muscles involved. The way in which the LOCUST works also has an excellent effect on the organs and glands located in the abdominal and groin areas. In the beginning you may have to struggle to raise your legs from the floor, but you will be surprised at how quickly you can regain control of these seldom-exercised muscles.

Points To Remember When Practicing the Locust

1. Your fists are placed with thumbs on the floor and your arms are drawn close in to your sides.

2. Fill your lungs only partly with air so that your chest is slightly expanded. If you inhale too deeply the posture becomes more difficult.

3. Keep your legs as straight as possible although you may bend your knees slightly if it helps you to raise your legs.

4. Keep your chin on the floor at all times; attempt to throw the weight of your lower body up to your arms and chin.

5. When the count is completed, lower your legs *slowly;* do not collapse. Allow the breath to be exhaled *slowly;* do not let it come rushing out. Always exhale through your nose.

YOUTH
**through *DYNAMIC CONVEX*
*STRETCHING AND STRENGTHENING***

● Technique No. 16—BOW

What the Bow Does for You

1. Relieves tension and develops the entire back through a powerful *convex* stretching movement.

2. Develops the chest and bust.

3. Helps to reduce weight in the abdomen, hips and thighs.

4. Aids in improving and maintaining a correct posture.

How To Do the Bow

The BOW always follows the LOCUST

1. When you have finished the LOCUST and are once again lying on your abdomen with your cheek resting on the floor and your arms at your sides, you are ready to perform the BOW.

2. Turn your head to rest your chin on the floor as in the LOCUST.

3. *Slowly* bend your legs at your knees and bring your feet up toward your back.

4. Reach back easily with your arms and carefully take hold of both feet. (You may grasp one foot first and then the other if easier.) You may have to struggle a moment to accomplish this. Once you are able to hold your feet, make sure your chin is on the floor. (Fig. 35)

5. Breathing normally (the breath is not held), attempt now to raise first your knees and then your trunk from the floor as far as possible *without strain*. Keep your head back and try to bring your knees together. Hold for the prescribed number of seconds. (Fig. 36)

6. *Slowly* come out of the posture as follows: first lower your knees to touch the floor; next allow your chin to touch the floor. Finally, release your feet and return them *slowly* to the floor. Rest your arms back at your sides. Thus you come out of the posture exactly the reverse of having gone into it.

7. Rest your cheek on the floor and relax.

Fig. 35

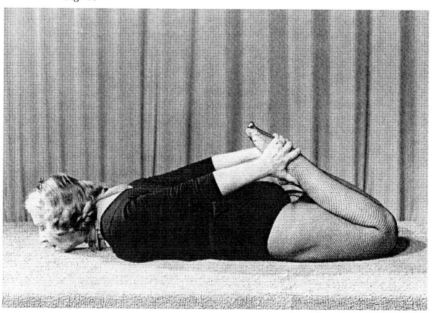

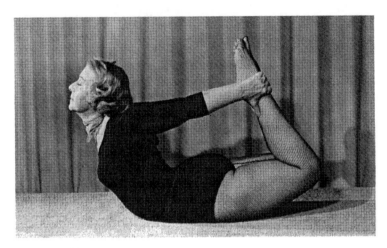

Fig. 36

How To Practice the Bow

Time to hold the extreme position:	begin with 10 seconds; add the seconds as advised in future weeks until 15 seconds are reached.
Number of times:	3; once following each LOCUST
Time of the day:	PM

Important Things To Know About the Bow

The BOW is the last of the great *convex* stretching and strengthening postures which bends the spine inward (as the COBRA and the LOCUST). It places strong emphasis on the entire back and especially the lumbar region. If you have been practicing as instructed, you should now be able to have at least partial success with this technique. You may, at first, have some difficulty in grasping both feet. If this is the case, you should reach easily for one foot first and then slowly try to work back to hold the other foot. You can lift your head back to aid you. Sometimes it requires a few attempts before you are successfully able to hold both feet. Next, you will probably be able to raise your trunk some distance from the floor even in your first try, but getting the knees and legs off the floor is often difficult because of the weakness of the muscles involved. However, if you can raise only your chest a few inches from the floor you will be strengthening, toning and relieving tension in your back. Repeated attempts will gradually build the strength necessary in the weakened muscles to lift your knees and thighs from the floor.

Points To Remember When Practicing the Bow

1. Make all of your movements slowly and cautiously, as this is a very powerful stretch.

2. If you have difficulty in grasping your feet, you may lift your head to aid you in reaching back farther. But once you are holding your feet, make sure that your chin comes back to the floor so that you are in the position of Fig. 35.

3. It is important to keep your head back when lifting your trunk and legs from the floor as described in step 5. (Fig. 36)

4. Breathe normally in the extreme position. Do not hold your breath.

5. When you raise your knees and thighs in the first attempts it may be easier for you to keep your knees some distance apart. But as you continue to gain strength, bring your knees together.

6. Come out of the BOW very slowly, exactly as instructed. Make sure that your knees touch first, then your chin; only when your chin is resting once again on the floor do you let go, *easily*, of your feet and return them *slowly* to the floor.

The 16 techniques you have now learned are grouped below under 'A,' 'B' and 'C.'

There are 2 methods of practicing these groups. Choose that method which you find most suitable.

> *Method 1*—Practice *twice* each day. Do group A in the AM and group B in the PM of the first day. Do group A in the AM and group C in the PM of the second day. On the third day, repeat the routine of the first day by doing group A in the AM and group B in the PM. On the fourth practice day, repeat the routine of the second day by doing group A in the AM and group C in the PM. On the fifth day, repeat the routine of the first day by doing group A in the AM and group B in the PM. Continue to alternate.

> *Method 2*—Practice *once* each day. Do group A the first day; do group B the second day; do group C the third day; do group A the fourth day, etc. Keep a record of your practice days on a separate sheet of paper so that you always know the correct group to do.

If the time given to hold a posture seems too difficult for you, you may modify the plan in accordance with your ability.

Practice very easily whenever you are stiff.

If you are not certain of how to do any of the movements of a particular technique, go back and read the instructions of that technique again. It is very important that you learn the techniques correctly.

Group A

No.	Name	Times	Hold
1	PRELIMINARY LEG PULL	3	20 sec°
2	KNEE AND THIGH STRETCH	3	15 sec°
3	BACKWARD BEND	2 feet	15 sec
		1 toes	15 sec
4	TOE TWIST	2 both sides	15 sec
5	ARM AND LEG STRETCH	2 both sides	10 sec°
13	ABDOMINAL LIFT	20 (5x4)	approx. 3 sec each lift°
10	COMPLETE BREATH (seated in one of the Lotus postures)	5 - 10	inhale: 15 sec° retain: 10 sec° exhale: 15 sec°

Group B

No.	Name	Times	Hold
1	PRELIMINARY LEG PULL	3	20 sec°
8	COBRA	See Next Page	15 sec
9	NECK MOVEMENTS	See Next Page	20 sec each movement°
15	LOCUST	See Next Page	5 sec
16	BOW	See Next Page	10 sec
14	ALTERNATE NOSTRIL BREATHING (seated in one of the Lotus postures)	5 rounds	inhale: count of 8° retain: count of 8° exhale: count of 8°

The cobra, neck movements, locust and bow will be performed as a unit in the following manner: begin by doing the cobra once; this will be followed by doing the neck movements once; next do the locust once; finally do the bow once; then begin again with the cobra, etc. This entire group of 4 techniques will be performed 3 times, holding each posture for the number of seconds indicated. We will continue this plan in future weeks of practice.

Group C

No.	Name	Times	Hold
1	PRELIMINARY LEG PULL	3	20 seconds°
7	CHEST EXPANSION	2	backward: 5 sec° forward: 10 sec°
11	SHOULDER STAND	1	2 minutes
12	EYE EXERCISES (seated in one of the Lotus postures)	10 clockwise; 10 counter-clockwise	a fraction-of-a-second hold on each of the 12 numbers°
13	ABDOMINAL LIFT	20 (5x4)	approx. 3 seconds each lift°
14	ALTERNATE NOSTRIL BREATHING (seated in one of the Lotus postures)	5 rounds	inhale: count of 8° retain: count of 8° exhale: count of 8°

° This is the final duration for this technique. No additional time will be added.

Notes: Sit in one of the Lotus postures whenever you can during the day. Do the COMPLETE BREATH, ARM AND LEG STRETCH, CHEST EXPANSION and ALTERNATE NOSTRIL BREATHING at any time of the day when you desire relief from fatigue, tension, anxiety.

On the first and second days of this Sixth Week carefully learn the 2 techniques listed below. Continue to practice the 16 techniques you have already learned according to page 120.

17. ALTERNATE LEG PULL
18. PLOUGH

On the third day of this week turn to page 135 and being your practice according to the 'Practice Plan' for this Sixth Week.

YOUTH
for the *LEGS*

● Technique No. 17—ALTERNATE LEG PULL

What the Alternate Leg Pull Does for You

1. Greatly stretches and strengthens the tendons, ligaments and muscles of the legs and feet.

2. Reduces and prevents flabbiness in the abdomen and thighs.

3. Develops the back, especially in the lumbar and shoulder areas.

How To Do the Alternate Leg Pull

1. Sit on the floor with your legs extended straight out in front of you, feet together and backs of the knees touching the floor.

2. Bend your right leg at the knee and bring the foot toward you so that you can take hold of it with both hands.

3. Place the sole of your right foot against the upper inside of your left thigh, with the right heel drawn as close to your groin as is possible. (See this position of the right foot in Fig. 37.)

4. In slow-motion, bend forward and take hold of the most extreme part of your leg that you can hold comfortably. This may be your knee, calf, ankle or foot. (Fig. 37)

5. Bend your elbows outward slightly and holding onto

your leg with your hands, pull gently and slowly forward, lowering your forehead as close to your left knee as possible. Do not strain. Make sure that the back of your left knee is touching the floor. Breathe slowly and close your eyes. Remain without motion in your extreme position for the prescribed time. (Fig. 38)

6. Release your hold on your leg and *slowly* raise your trunk to the upright position. Rest several moments and repeat.

7. When you have completed your movements with your left leg, slowly extend the right leg straight out before you. Now bend the *left* leg at the knee and bring it toward you so that you can take hold of your left foot with both hands. Proceed exactly as in step 3, simply substituting the word "left" for "right" and vice-versa.

Fig. 37

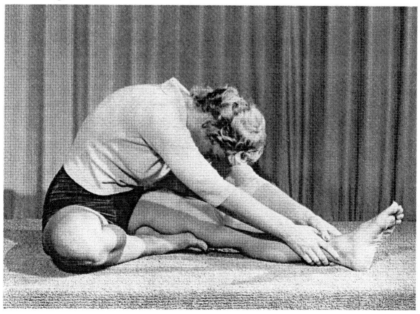

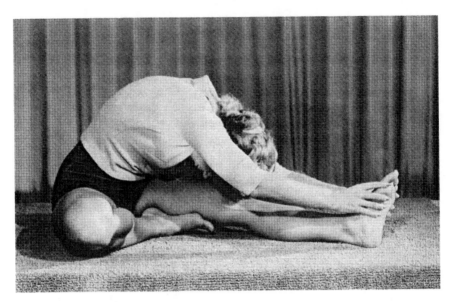

Fig. 38

How To Practice the Alternate Leg Pull

Time to hold the extreme position:	begin with 20 seconds for each movement; add the seconds as advised in future weeks until 30 seconds are reached.
Number of times:	2 times for each leg
Time of the day:	PM

Important Things To Know About the Alternate Leg Pull

This technique is designed to stretch and strengthen the legs individually. The movement is similar to our first technique, the PRELIMINARY LEG PULL, with the exception that here we practice first with one leg and then the other. The principle is the same: go only as far as you can and hold your extreme position motionless. This will enable you to get down farther each day. When you are working with your *left* leg you will find the lower *right* part of your back is being greatly stretched. The converse is true of the opposite side. If this posture seems to cause a great pull in the beginning, it is because you have grown stiff and tense throughout your legs and back. The ALTER-NATE LEG PULL is another excellent technique to aid you in eliminating energy-sapping tension as well as put new "spring" into your back and legs.

Points To Remember When Practicing the Alternate Leg Pull

1. Keep the back of the knee of your outstretched leg touching the floor. It does not matter how far down you are able to hold your leg in the beginning. But if you bend your leg at the knee in order to reach farther forward, you will lose the real stretch.

2. Always aim your forehead down toward your knee. Allow your neck to go limp.

3. Remember to bend your elbows slightly outward. This aids in the stretch.

4. Close your eyes; breathe slowly; count the seconds silently to yourself.

YOUTH
through *DYNAMIC CONCAVE STRETCHING AND STRENGTHENING*

● Technique No. 18—PLOUGH

What the Plough Does for You

1. Develops great elasticity in the spine.

2. Greatly strengthens the back, abdomen and neck.

3. Relieves tension throughout these areas.

4. Helps to reduce weight in the legs, thighs, hips and abdomen and firms the muscles and skin of these areas.

How To Do the Plough

1. Lie flat on your back with your arms at your sides. Allow your body to go limp; close your eyes; breathe normally.

2. Turn your palms downward so that they press against the floor. Bring your legs together and tense your leg and abdominal muscles.

3. *Slowly* raise your legs up into the air until they are at a right angle with the floor.

4. Keep your knees stiff; press down hard on the floor with your palms; swing your legs easily back over your head.

5. Continue to push down on the floor with your hands and keep your knees straight. *Slowly* lower your legs behind you as far toward the floor as possible. Stop at whatever point this movement becomes a strain and

simply hold your extreme position for the prescribed number of seconds. Close your eyes and breathe slowly. (Fig. 39) The ultimate position is reached when your feet touch the floor and your knees remain straight. (Fig. 40)

6. To come out of this posture, bend your legs at the knees and bring the knees close to your head. (Fig. 41) Now roll forward and arch your neck so that you can keep the back of your head and your upper back on the floor.

7. When your back is resting on the floor, extend your legs straight out into the air and slowly lower them to the floor.

8. Allow your body to go completely limp and rest for at least 1 minute.

Fig. 39

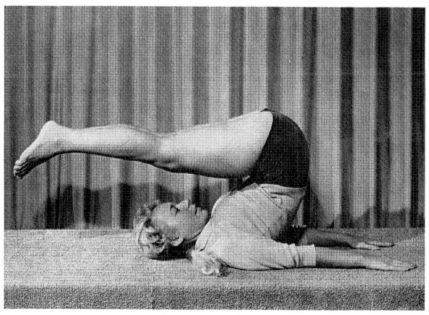

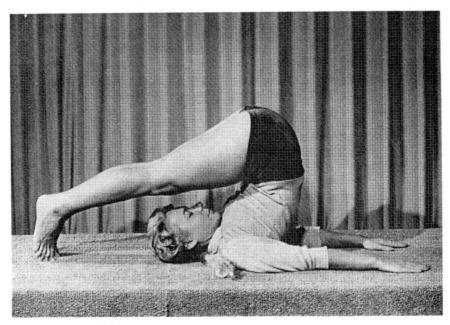

Fig. 40

How To Practice the Plough

Time to hold the extreme position:	begin with 20 seconds; add the seconds as advised in future weeks until you reach 30 seconds.
Number of times:	2
Time of the day:	PM

Important Things To Know About the Plough

The PLOUGH is an advanced stretching posture which you should now be able to perform with some success. Just as the BOW was a powerful *convex* (inward) posture, so is the PLOUGH a dynamic *concave* (outward) posture.

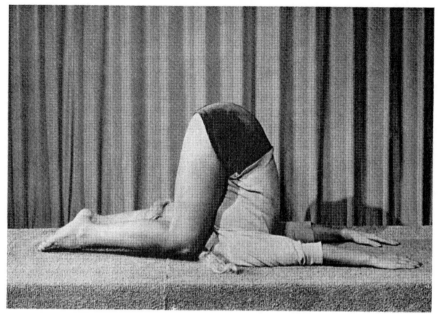

Fig. 41

It greatly streamlines and strengthens the back and spine as well as the legs. Of course you must begin by going back only as far as you are able to and simply holding your extreme position so that the vertebrae slowly work out and you are gradually able to drop your feet another inch or two toward the floor. There is no point in straining to accomplish the extreme position because if you cannot do it comfortably, it is an obvious indication that your spine is stiff and that you must work out the stiffness slowly. Gradually you will feel that the pressure changes from the base of your spine in your first attempts, to the middle of your spine as you continue to practice, and finally, when you are able to place your toes well behind your head on the floor, you will feel the emphasis in your upper back and neck.

Points To Remember When Practicing the Plough

1. Do not strain or force the position. Just go as far back as you are able to and maintain your extreme position for the necessary number of seconds. Your legs will automatically drop a little farther each day.

2. Keep your legs straight at all times when going back. Try not to bend your knees.

3. Close your eyes and count the seconds silently; breathe slowly.

4. Come out of the posture with control and grace as instructed.

5. Rest in the reclining position for at least 30 seconds.

The 18 techniques you have now learned are grouped below under 'A,' 'B' and 'C.'

There are 2 methods of practicing these groups. These methods are described on page 120. Choose that method which you find most suitable.

If the time given to hold a posture seems too difficult for you, you may modify the plan in accordance with your ability.

Practice very easily whenever you are stiff.

If you are not certain of how to do any of the movements of a particular technique, go back and read the instructions of that technique again. It is very important that you learn the techniques correctly.

Group A

No.	Name	Times	Hold
1	PRELIMINARY LEG PULL	3	20 sec°
2	KNEE AND THIGH STRETCH	3	15 sec°
3	BACKWARD BEND	2 feet 1 toes	20 sec° 20 sec°
4	TOE TWIST	2 both sides	15 sec
5	ARM AND LEG STRETCH	2 both sides	10 sec°
13	ABDOMINAL LIFT	25 (5x5)	approx. 3 seconds each lift°
10	COMPLETE BREATH (seated in one of the Lotus postures)	5 - 10	inhale: 15 sec° retain: 10 sec° exhale: 15 sec°

Group B

No.	Name	Times	Hold
1	PRELIMINARY LEG PULL	3	20 sec°
8	COBRA	⎤	20 sec°
9	NECK MOVEMENTS	⎬ To be practiced as indicated on page 122.	20 seconds each movement°
15	LOCUST		7 sec
16	BOW	⎦	12 sec
11	SHOULDER STAND	1	2½ minutes
14	ALTERNATE NOSTRIL BREATHING (seated in one of the Lotus postures)	5 rounds	inhale: count of 8° retain: count of 8° exhale: count of 8°

Group C

No.	Name	Times	Hold
1	PRELIMINARY LEG PULL	3	20 sec°
7	CHEST EXPANSION	2	backward: 5 sec° forward: 10 sec°
12	EYE EXERCISES (seated in one of the Lotus postures)	10 clockwise; 10 counter-clockwise	a fraction of a second hold on each of the 12 numbers°
13	ABDOMINAL LIFT	25 (5x5)	approx. 3 seconds each lift°
17	ALTERNATE LEG PULL	2 each leg	20 sec
18	PLOUGH	2	20 sec
14	ALTERNATE NOSTRIL BREATHING (seated in one of the Lotus postures)	5 rounds	inhale: count of 8° retain: count of 8° exhale: count of 8°

° This is the final duration for this technique. No additional time will be added.

Notes: Sit in one of the Lotus postures whenever you can during the day. Do the COMPLETE BREATH, ARM AND LEG STRETCH, CHEST EXPANSION and ALTERNATE NOSTRIL BREATHING at any time of the day when you desire relief from fatigue, tension, anxiety.

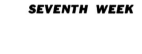

SEVENTH WEEK

On the first and second days of this Seventh Week carefully learn the 2 techniques listed below. Continue to practice the 18 techniques you have already learned according to page 135.

19.   COMPLETE LEG PULL
20.   HEAD STAND

On the third day of this week turn to page 148 and begin your "Complete Plan of Practice."

YOUTH
through *COMPLETE ELASTICITY*
OF THE SPINE

● Technique No. 19—COMPLETE LEG PULL

What the Complete Leg Pull Does for You

1. Provides complete elasticity for the spine.

2. Greatly develops and tones the back with a dynamic *concave* stretching movement.

3. Strengthens the entire leg and makes the skin taut and firm.

How To Do the Complete Leg Pull

1. We will perform the COMPLETE LEG PULL following the PLOUGH. From the reclining position of the PLOUGH slowly raise your trunk to a sitting position. As you are doing this, extend your arms straight out before you.

2. *Slowly* bend your trunk forward and have your extended hands grasp the farthermost area of your legs that you can hold. (Fig. 42)

3. Bend your elbows outward and *slowly* pull your trunk forward and downward. Lower your forehead to rest as close to your knees as possible. Hold your extreme position for the prescribed number of seconds. The ultimate stretching posture, with the elbows touching the floor and the hands holding the feet, is illustrated in Fig. 43.

4. Release your legs and *slowly* return to the sitting position.

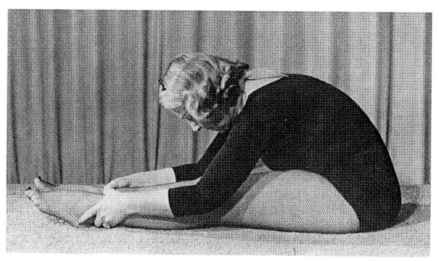

Fig. 42

How To Practice the Complete Leg Pull

Time to hold the extreme
position: begin with 25 seconds; add
                                   the seconds as advised until
                                   30 seconds are reached.
Number of times: 2
Time of the day: PM

Fig. 43

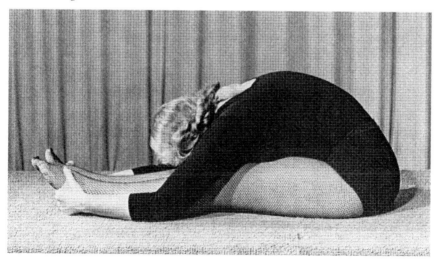

Important Things To Know About the Complete Leg Pull

The COMPLETE LEG PULL is the last of the intense *concave* stretches. It is actually the complimentary exercise to the PLOUGH and will be performed following the PLOUGH. You will notice the similarity between this posture and the very first technique, the PRELIMINARY LEG PULL. However, there is an important distinction: the PRELIMINARY LEG PULL is a *preparatory* movement, practiced very gently to help work out the stiffness and tenseness, especially in the early morning. The COMPLETE LEG PULL, which is performed in the PM, when you have already loosened your spine, is a much more advanced technique in which you make a real attempt to reach very far down with your hands and lower your head almost to your knees. As such, there is the ultimate stretching of both the back and legs as you can see from the illustrations. There is no "trick" or strain involved in this movement. Your spine simply loosens to such an extent that gradually complete elasticity results. You will accomplish this if you follow the instructions for practice and you will notice a great difference in your appearance and the way you feel when you have gained this wonderful elasticity.

Points To Remember When Practicing the Complete Leg Pull

1. As you reach down with your hands, bend your feet back toward you and you may be able to hold your toes.

2. Keep the backs of your knees on the floor and your legs together; remember to bend your elbows outward and allow your neck to go limp; close your eyes; breathe slowly; count the seconds silently.

YOUTH
through *REVITALIZING*
THE BRAIN

● Technique No. 20—HEAD STAND

What the Head Stand Does for You

1. Restores vitality and activates the nerve centers in the brain.

2. Improves the faculties of the brain; maintains alertness of mind.

3. Helps to prevent and stop falling hair.

4. Often improves vision and hearing.

How To Do the Head Stand

1. Sit on your heels as we began the BACKWARD BEND. Keep your knees together on the floor.

2. Interlace your fingers and place your clasped hands and forearms on the floor in front of you.

3. Place the top of your head on the floor and hold the back of your head with your clasped hands. (Fig. 44)

4. Raise your trunk and knees from the floor so that you are on your toes and forming the arch as in Fig. 45.

5. Walk forward on your toes until you have brought your knees as close to your chest as possible. (Fig. 45)

6. Now it is a question of pushing off from the floor lightly with your toes and transferring the weight so that it is evenly distributed between your head and forearms.

Keep your legs folded and close in to your chest. (Fig. 46) *Go no farther until you have mastered this position.* Hold for the prescribed number of seconds and return your feet lightly to the floor.

7. To complete the HEAD STAND, *slowly* straighten your legs once you have mastered the above position until your body is in a vertical position. (Figs. 47, 48, 49) Hold for the prescribed period of time. (Fig. 50 depicts a variation in the HEAD STAND.)

8. To come out of the posture, fold your legs at the knees so that you return slowly to the floor in the exact reverse manner of having gone up. Always keep the knees close to the body.

9. Rest on the floor with your head down for at least 1 minute.

10. *Slowly* sit up into the Lotus, or cross-legged, posture.

How To Practice the Head Stand

Time to hold the extreme position:

begin with 30 seconds; add the seconds as advised in the *COMPLETE PLAN OF PRACTICE* until 3 minutes are reached. You can eventually hold this 5 minutes and longer as desired.

Number of times: 1

Time of the day: PM

Important Things To Know About the Head Stand

The HEAD STAND offers the most effective method to refresh the brain. In addition to this, its other therapeutic

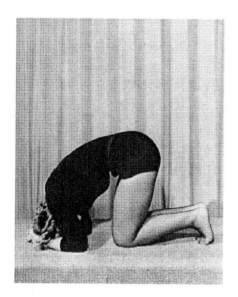

Fig. 44

Fig. 45

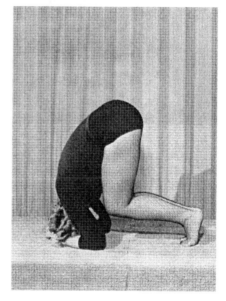

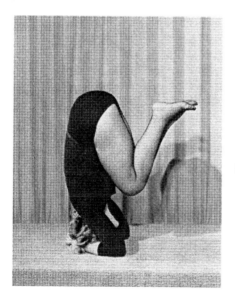

Fig. 46

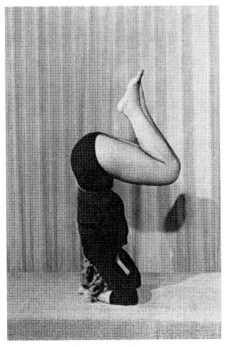
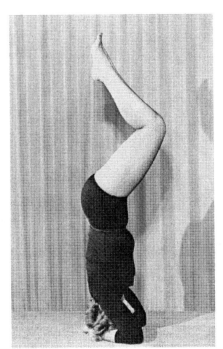

Fig. 47   *Fig. 48*

values make it a highly valuable technique to master. Most people quickly gain the balance necessary for the HEAD STAND either under their own power or with the aid of the wall. Do the HEAD STAND on a fairly soft surface (such as a rug or carpet) so that if you lose your balance you will not be bruised. Also, it is best to place a pillow directly beneath your head to help take the pressure off your neck. If your neck is uncomfortable after doing the HEAD STAND, allow several days to elapse before you do it again. You must never experience any continual strain. If you want to use the wall for help, then place your head a foot or two from the wall and as you raise your body, allow the feet to come forward and rest against the wall. In this way you can slowly "walk" up the wall and then try to gently "push" your feet from the wall and maintain your balance. Repeated attempts will bring success. Do not neglect this posture.

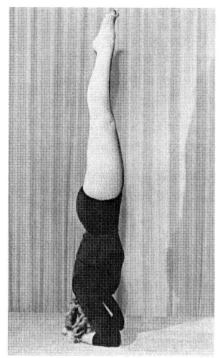
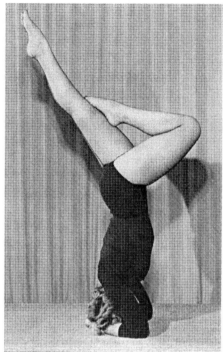

Fig. 49   Fig. 50

Points To Remember When Practicing the Head Stand

1. Always "walk" in and bring your knees as close to your chest as possible. This makes it easy to control the shifting of weight.

2. Make sure you master the first position before attempting to straighten up all the way.

3. Place a watch or clock in a position where you can glance at it.

4. Once mastered, close your eyes and breathe slowly in the inverted posture.

5. Come out of the posture slowly, with control; do not drop to the floor suddenly. Relax with your head down for at least 1 minute.

You have now learned the complete course of 20 techniques. These 20 techniques are grouped below in a 'complete plan of practice. You may use this plan to remain fit and youthful for your entire life.

There are 2 methods for practice which have already been described on page 89. Choose that method which you find most suitable.

Continue to practice patiently and carefully, following all directions as closely as possible. You will experience wonderful results quickly.

You have begun your journey on the road to a second youth!

Group A

No.	Name	Times	Hold
1	PRELIMINARY LEG PULL	3	20 sec°
2	KNEE AND THIGH STRETCH	3	15 sec°
3	BACKWARD BEND	2 feet	20 sec°
		1 toes	20 sec°
4	TOE TWIST	2 both sides (left-right; left-right)	20 sec°
5	ARM AND LEG STRETCH	2 both sides (2 with left arm; 2 with right arm)	10 sec°

Group A (con't)

No.	Name	Times	Hold
13	ABDOMINAL LIFT	25-50 (done in groups of 5 to 10)	approx. 3 seconds each lift°
10	COMPLETE BREATH (seated in one of the Lotus postures)	5-10	inhale: 15 sec° retain: 10 sec° exhale: 15 sec° ———————— THIS ROUTINE REQUIRES APPROXI- MATELY 20 MINUTES

Group B

No.	Name	Times	Hold
1	PRELIMINARY LEG PULL	3	20 sec°
8	COBRA	Read informa-	20 sec°
9	NECK MOVEMENTS	tion relating to these 4	20 seconds each movement°
15	LOCUST	postures on	10 sec°
16	BOW	page 122.	15 sec°
11	SHOULDER STAND	1	3 minutes° (you may hold this posture for 5 minutes and longer as desired)
14	ALTERNATE NOS- TRIL BREATHING (seated in one of the Lotus postures)	5 rounds	inhale: count of 8° retain: count of 8° exhale: count of 8° ———————— THIS ROUTINE REQUIRES AP- PROXIMATELY 30 MINUTES

Group C

No.	Name	Times	Hold
7	CHEST EXPANSION	2	backward: 5 sec° forward: 10 sec°
12	EYE EXERCISES (seated on one of the Lotus postures)	10 clockwise; 10 counter-clockwise	a fraction-of-a-second hold on each of the 12 numbers°
17	ALTERNATE LEG PULL	These 3 techniques will be	30 sec°
18	PLOUGH	practiced as	30 sec° (after having practiced
19	COMPLETE LEG PULL	a unit in the manner described below	technique for 2 days with 25 seconds, you may now hold for 30)
20	HEAD STAND	1	30 seconds. This is the only technique in which you will have to add time at the rate of 30 seconds per week until 3 minutes are reached. You can eventually hold this posture for 5 minutes and longer as desired.
14	ALTERNATE NOS-TRIL BREATHING (seated in one of the Lotus postures)	5 rounds	inhale: count of 8° retain: count of 8° exhale: count of 8°
			THIS ROUTINE REQUIRES APPROXIMATELY 30 MINUTES

° This is the final duration for this technique.

The alternate leg pull, plough and complete leg pull will be performed as a unit in the following manner: begin by doing the alternate leg pull once with each leg; next lie on your back and perform the plough once; finally do the complete leg pull once. Then begin again and repeat the exact same routine. Thus you will have performed each of these techniques twice.

Notes: Sit in one of the Lotus postures whenever you can during the day. Do the COMPLETE BREATH, ARM AND LEG STRETCH, CHEST EXPANSION and ALTERNATE NOSTRIL BREATH-ING at any time of the day when you desire relief from fatigue, tension, anxiety.

Part II

This section contains important details of the charactertistics of 'Youth and Age' as they appear on page 5. Here we will deal with problems which may arise from these categories through specific routines of the exercises. You should complete the seven weeks of practice and perform the 'Complete Plan of Practice' for at least four weeks exactly as indicated before you devote additional practice time to the special routines listed in this section.

1. FLEXIBILITY AND GRACE;
Stretching Your Way to Beauty

YOUTH	AGE
Flexibility—suppleness— agility; grace—poise— balance	Stiffness—tightness— immobility; awkwardness— lack of poise

Usually the first physical characteristics of which we become aware when we see someone is his or her *movements* and *posture*. The way in which a person moves, gestures, walks, sits and stands actually makes a strong impression upon us. Isn't it true that if a person, regardless of age, moves with a certain spring and agility that he appears youthful and alive? Is there not something magnetic and radiant about the man or woman who walks, stands and sits with natural grace and poise? And on the other hand, how quickly we will regard as "old" those people who have allowed their spines and limbs to grow stiff. Stiffness and tightness will always lead to varying degrees of immobility, slumping, stooping and awkwardness and we seem to be instinctively repelled by these characteristics which detract from what should be the natural beauty of the body.

Flexibility, balance and poise are not characteristics which can be "faked." That is, you cannot *force* a good posture or move with grace and agility if you don't really feel these naturally. But in reality the body is the temple of the spirit; therefore, it *is* the natural condition of the human body to have the attributes of youth and beauty and it is only through neglect that they are lost. We can regain them as we stimulate and increase the vital force through the Yoga exercises.

The major offenders from the standpoint of stiffness, tightness and resulting lack of agility and poise are the spine and · back. The joints also play a major role. Let us first make a few important observations from the Yogic viewpoint regarding the spine. The Yogi will tell you that you feel and look as young as your spine is elastic. You have only to look at the people around you to determine the truth of this idea. Your friends and relatives who may be young in years will appear to be "aging" as their spines and joints stiffen and they find it increasingly difficult to accomplish the necessary tasks of everyday life, let alone moving their bodies with agility and poise. On the other hand you will find a certain "ageless" quality in that person who, regardless of age in years, has maintained the elasticity of his spine. He walks, moves and bends with ease and grace; he appears poised and agile and as such is bound to radiate the characteristics of youth, health and even optimism, attributes which we find so positive and attractive.

The spine is a structure which must have continual and *methodical* exercise. You may remember that we have compared the spine to a jack-in-the-box. Unless it receives the proper care it will gradually be compressed and squeezed into a smaller and smaller area. This is what happens to most people as they grow older, for they fail to stretch and manipulate the spine and it grows increasingly stiff and actually constricts. The stiffer the spine becomes the more inactive one grows and the more inactive, the stiffer the spine. This vicious circle can, however, be broken when one begins to manipulate his spine through the gentle practices of Yoga. The spine begins to stretch out once again and the elasticity which the spine can regain as the lid is removed from the jack-in-the-box is truly amazing. Remember that this is true regardless of age.

It is interesting to note that the entire science of therapy through chiropractic is based on manipulation of the various areas of the spine and of the joints. It is the theory of the chiropractor that every function of the body is in some way related to the spinal structure and that the incorrect position of the vertebrae in the spine can be responsible for illnesses throughout the organism. To relieve the pressure of one group of vertebrae from pressing upon another or to correct the position of individual vertebrae, the chiropractor administers "adjustments" to the spine. Similarly, the yogi attaches great value to a strong, elastic spine and many of our Yoga exercises are practiced for the express purpose of promoting the health, strength and flexibility of the entire spine, from the cervical vertebrae in the neck to the lowest of the vertebrae in the lumbar area.

In connection with this type of manipulation I should like to state that it is my opinion that many cases of arthritis could be prevented or kept from spreading in the body through the serious, careful, patient practice of Yoga. I say this because of my experience with many thousands of Yoga students. Although I have never prescribed the Yoga exercises for any illness or disease and always insist that a prospective Yoga student who has a history of illness first consult his physician before undertaking any exercise, the percentage of students who have reported to me that they have experienced a noticeable relief of their arthritic discomforts cannot be ignored.* You may be aware that arthritis is an illness in which the sufferer seldom improves. If he is fortunate, the pain is kept to a minimum through medical treatment and the disease is localized to one part of the body. More generally, however, arthritis *does* slowly spread and the pain becomes gradually more intense. I believe that what accounts for the relief of arthritic symptoms through the Yoga techniques is the *thoroughness* of the exercises; these slow-motion movements and "holds," unlike ordinary forms of exercise, are able to reach

---

* This is certainly noteworthy in light of current statistics. Dr. Alexander Goodman, president of the Arthritis National Research Foundation (Los Angeles) has informed me that there are now approximately 15,000,000 Americans afflicted with arthritis and rheumatism and that this number is expected to double to 30,000,000 by 1964!

deeply into the stiff joints. The methodical repetition of these movements, practiced very easily and slowly, and even discontinued on days when real discomfort is present, seems within the course of time to produce some very wonderful results. If you are an arthritic you should certainly consult your physician regarding the practice of Yoga, and if you receive his consent you should stress the exercises presented at the end of this chapter. You must practice very carefully and seriously and keep in mind that it has taken you many years to develop this painful disease and it would be highly unrealistic to expect an overnight miracle. All improvement in nature is *progressive*.

The Yoga spinal exercises have still another important implication. From the Yogic viewpoint, in addition to the normal energies and impulses which should flow freely from the body to the brains through the healthy spine, there are powerful energies which are asleep, untapped within the spine. These energies form part of the vital force which we are awakening through all of our Yoga techniques. It is the premise of *Kundalini* Yoga that this great reservoir of energy within the spine (and certain other areas, known as "centers," of the organism) can be tapped and used. You are certain to notice the all-day "bounce" and "spring" that you have as this extra force becomes available to you.

Regarding the back, it is curious how many Americans suffer needlessly with stiffness, tightness and other discomforts in the various areas of the back. The areas usually involved in most complaints are the back of the shoulders and the lower back throughout the lumbar region. Massages, steam, linaments offer only temporary relief; again methodical, nonstrenuous stretching and strengthening is the Yogic solution to these problems. There is hardly an occupation which does not present a hazard in some degree to the back. Persons who work at a desk, drivers, construction workers, housewives, all place continual stress on particular areas of the back and many of these workers who are always complaining about the discomforts which are certain to result from this continual stress are unaware that daily relief is possible through the simple process of methodical stretching. It is necessary to note once again that there is a confusion in the minds of many people between "activity" and "exercise." The housewife or construction worker may scoff at the idea of exercising or manipulating the body since they mistakenly believe that they have had plenty of activity during the workday and that what they should do after their work is completed is rest. This is true to a certain extent but rest will not actually work out stiffness and discomfort. It is not the *amount* of activity or movement that keeps the body healthy and flexible; it is the *type* of movement. Most of the activity of the housewife, for example, creates conditions of stress. Her movements cannot correctly be considered as exercise since most of these movements will promote stiffness and stress, not relieve them. The same is true for the farmer or the man who thinks that he is getting plenty of exercise by working in his garden. He will usually finish his chores having *produced* conditions of stress and strain. Perhaps the most curious of all of the examples which I could give you along these lines is the person who believes that he is receiving the necessary exercise and maintaining his health and flexibility by engaging in one or more of the popular sports. Golf, bowling, tennis, horseback riding and fishing can certainly be enjoyable, and participating in any or all of these is infinitely better than not being active at all. However, it is a fallacy to believe that these sports, which make use of only specific sets of muscles in repetitious, quick, sudden, forceful and often strenuous movements, can be expected to maintain the true suppleness and flexibility of spine, joints and limbs that is our objective in Yoga. I am always inclined to smile inwardly when a student who begins the practice of Yoga informs me that he has remained "fit" by playing 18 holes of golf each Sunday and Wednesday. He may have a suntanned exterior, but when he begins the first Yoga stretches he realizes to his surprise that his back and spine are as stiff as a board. Indeed, going a step further, some of the stiffest, most inflexible people I have ever encountered in my classes are amateur or professional athletes! Their muscles are frequently overdeveloped, cramped, stiff, tight; they are afflicted with continual sprains, slipped discs, charleyhorses; they must work out constantly in the most frightfully strenuous routines to keep their muscles from turning into fat. In this connection, I believe it is a fundamental error in the physical education program of our schools to so overemphasize and glamorize the merits of sports, rather than stress the learning of intelligent routines which a student could continue to follow after leaving school and throughout his entire life for maintaining true health of body and mind. Such routines would indeed become the basis for a realistic national physical fitness program. You may be interested to know that among my students, I have found that those who have engaged in a moderate routine of swimming and walking have maintained the greatest flexibility. Swimming can be considered to be the finest sport because, as in Yoga, so many areas of the body are used in rhythmic, coordinated and often slow-motion movements. Also, almost all of the girls and women who have studied ballet at one time or another seem to have benefited greatly from the standpoint of flexibility, grace, poise and balance.

I believe you will agree that grace, poise and balance are also important characteristics of youth and beauty. These attributes grow out of suppleness and flexibility. You cannot move gracefully and have the posture necessary to radiate poise and a sense of balance and control of your body if your spine and joints are stiff. It is truly remarkable how Yoga students feel and look years younger simply by regaining their ability to pull in their abdomens and walk with their shoulders back and their spines straight. This improvement takes place in a most natural manner when the spine once again becomes supple. It seems that as the spine loosens, the trunk will automatically want to straighten and one cannot help but begin to move gracefully. Also, stretching and developing the arms and legs as we do with the Yoga exercises greatly aids in this process. A wonderful sense of control and balance is developed by mastering the TOE TWIST, ARM and LEG STRETCH, ALTERNATE LEG PULL, SHOULDER STAND and HEAD STAND postures.

It often happens that when people who have been practicing Yoga meet friends whom they have not seen for some time, a frequent comment is something such as, "What have you been doing? You look different but I don't know exactly what it is." The "difference" is a subtle one, due largely to the flexibility and resulting poise which has been gained through the Yoga exercises. These subtle characteristics cannot fail to be felt by anyone who comes in contact with them. Regardless of what you do during the day remind yourself to do it with grace and poise. The slogan is: "Think gracefully!" If you "think gracefully" you find that you will move and act gracefully. This very quickly becomes a habit and carries over into all of your activities. Every type of work can then assume dignity and be accomplished with much greater ease. It is a wonderful thing to feel this metamorphosis; it is truly a rebirth!

Here are the techniques to be emphasized for:

Flexibility—Suppleness—Agility; Grace—Poise—Balance

According to your needs regarding a specific problem you can emphasize the techniques listed below as they appear in your COMPLETE PLAN OF PRACTICE for that particular day. The word "emphasize" implies that you could add additional seconds gradually to the Practice Plan and you could slowly increase the repetitions by two or three. If you prefer you can practice the indicated routine separately from your regular Practice Plan but in the event that you stress certain techniques, do not do so at the expense of neglecting your COMPLETE PLAN OF PRACTICE. If you undertake to practice any one or group of exercises more intensely, always do so with restraint and intelligence, as there must never be any straining or forcing in Yoga.

FLEXIBILITY–Spine

Leg Pulls	(1)	(19)
Backward Bend	(3)	
Toe Twist	(4)	
Chest Expansion	(7)	
Cobra	(8)	
Plough	(18)	

FLEXIBILITY–Neck

Neck Movements	(9)
Shoulder Stand	(11)
Plough	(18)

FLEXIBILITY–Toes, Feet, Ankles, Knees

Knee and Thigh Stretch	(2)
Backward Bend	(3)
Toe Twist	(4)
Lotus Postures	(6)

Grace–Poise–Balance

Toe Twist	(4)
Arm and Leg Stretch	(5)
Shoulder Stand	(11)
Alternate Leg Pull	(17)
Head Stand	(20)

FLEXIBILITY–Elbows, Shoulders

Backward Bend	(3)
Toe Twist	(4)
Arm and Leg Stretch	(5)
Chest Expansion	(7)

POSTURE

Backward Bend	(3)
Arm and Leg Stretch	(5)
Chest Expansion	(7)
Cobra	(8)
Bow	(16)
Plough	(18)

2. TENSION;
Exposing the Multiheaded Dragon

YOUTH	*AGE*
Ability to relax as necessary —calmness—composure— serenity; restful sleep.	Tension—nervousness— irritability—poor disposi- tion; insomnia.

How often have you heard the following: "You must relax," or "Try to be calm," or "Get a grip on yourself"? If you think about these expressions for a few moments you will detect an obvious contradiction. What is implied in these expressions is: *"Order* yourself to relax"; *"Command* yourself to be calm"; *"Try hard* to remain tranquil." But the very nature of relaxation, calmness and tranquility is directly opposed to ordering, commanding or trying hard. If you are trying hard to relax, how can you be relaxed? You are too busy trying! The essence of relaxation is to be free from the anxiety of "trying hard." In short, you cannot *make* yourself relax. It is impossible to force tranquility upon yourself.

Relaxation is a kind of physical and mental "letting go." This must come naturally and cannot be forced. Ideally, one should be able to maintain the "letting go" feeling at all times, for it is in this state that one's best work is done. All tasks are then accomplished easily, and you are probably aware that the less worry which goes into a job, the more successfully the job is done. But unfortunately most people consider relaxation as something which is supposed to be done at specific times. In other words, we set aside *periods* for relaxation. We decide that our ordinary work is hard, tedious, wearisome and for the most part uninteresting, and when the workday is over or the necessary chores are completed we then attempt to engage in some type of "relaxation." It is at such specified times that we try to "let go." But Americans are finding it more and more difficult to let go even when they are supposed to be relaxing and having a good time. This is because all of the anxious and irritating sensations and experiences that have piled up during the workday refuse to put on their collective hats and take a temporary leave on cue. This may be somewhat of an oversimplification but the crux of the matter is that we now find this terrible paradox among millions of people in our country: we are fighting desperately to let go. We are downing tons of tranquilizers and consuming oceans of alcoholic beverages; we are supposedly entertaining ourselves with the most horrendous junk on the screens and in print, all in a frantic effort to have some form of distraction or escape which we have confused with "relaxation." But the harder we fight to distract ourselves, the more impossible it becomes to relax. We have fallen into a peculiar trap of our own making.

The villain of the piece is a vague, shadowy figure hovering in the background and upon whose convenient head we have collectively lumped practically every cause of our inability to relax and to function harmoniously. This villain is well known to every American and strikes particular fear into the heart of the television viewer. The name of this culprit is TENSION! The word "tension" has been used in Part I of this book mostly in a physical context. But tension has come to mean many things to many people. Tension is the "anxiety" of the psychoanalyst; he is the "insecurity" of the breadwinner; he is the "life-shortener" of the statistician; he is the "case of nerves" of the physician; he is the "burned dinner" of the housewife; he appears as the hammer, chisel and electric drill in the television commercial; he is the "nervousness" of the athlete and performer; he is responsible for mass hysteria, bad disposition, poor golf scores, mob violence, stiff necks, sleepless nights and broken homes. And as though this were not bad enough, he has an even more ferocious big brother whose name is HYPERTENSION! Quite a formidable family! Let us go along with these concepts and presume that this monster, tension, *is* responsible for all of the above. How does one deal with this multiheaded dragon? Well, take heart, because through our practice of Yoga we will have developed several highly effective weapons for the battle.

First let us remark that there is certainly great stress from current world conditions; the disturbances are all about us and we cannot help but feel them. We do not mean to minimize this situation. But tension is today, as it has always been under different names, a highly individual and personal problem. In all of the continual social and political crises throughout human history there are always those who are able to maintain their composure, dignity and serenity, and as such, be of real aid to their fellow man. You can catch the fear (tension) of a nuclear war from your neighbor the same as you can catch his cold. But just as you can avoid catching his cold if your physical resistance is adequate, so can you avoid catching tensions if your level of serenity is sufficiently high. If, through the strength of your religious faith or philosophical beliefs you are not beset with tensions, then you may have no problem along these lines. You should probably be able to maintain your tranquility. But a vast number of our fellow Americans are suffering from the various forms of disturbances, anxiety and fear which are classified under the general term of "tension," and for them I should like to offer a routine of the Yoga practices which, throughout many centuries, have been used so successfully to achieve a high, natural level of tranquility. Through these Yoga practices you do not have to force yourself to relax; you do not have to fight to "let go." This happens effortlessly, naturally, beautifully.

The term "tension" is really quite vague and there are as many feelings and definitions about this as there are people who have experienced any type of disturbance or uneasiness. Of course, if tension manifests itself as an obvious physical or mental illness, one should not hesitate to seek competent medical advice. But for purposes of this discussion let us picture tension as a definite entity—as, let us say, a villain. We will find that our villain has all of the characteristics of a bully. You do not expose a bully by attempting to escape from him; no more can you expose the tyrannical nature of anxiety, fear, insecurity, apprehension and physical discomfort by seeking relief in the distractions and pacifiers which are so readily offered to us. You must face the bully and take bold and decisive action. Let us imagine that you are very much under the domination of a severe form of tension and that you expect momentarily to explode from its intensity. In other words, suppose that you have reached the absolute maximum of tension, exactly as may be the case a number of times each day. You must now do a very bold thing. You must stop running! Turn around and *welcome the tension.* Shake hands with him. Invite him in so that you may become better acquainted. Tell him that he is welcome to do whatever he wants and that you will offer no resistance. This is the first step at exposure, at turning the light on him. He will be so startled at this turn of events that he will be temporarily neutralized. The wind will be taken out of his sails and the force of his feared punch will be greatly diminished. But you cannot fake this welcome. You must bravely and genuinely offer him whatever he wants. In essence, you are asking him to do his worst and you are prepared to accept whatever this may be. This is the last thing in the world he could have expected. To your great surprise, it may be that, like a bully, he has never really wanted a fight. All he wanted to do was to scare you and as long as he succeeded in keeping you in a state of fear and uneasiness he has accomplished his purpose. Now, however, you are standing up to him and politely calling his bluff.

Next, while you are extending your gentle invitation, you undertake a number of the Yoga practices as outlined at the end of this chapter. These techniques are extremely dynamic and there is nothing more powerful that you could do to cope with the dragons of tension in a natural manner. Gradually through this method you should be able to overcome all forms of tension. You may have to repeat some part or all of this program several times each day or whenever relief of the symptoms of tension is needed. But it is possible to work with certain of the calming techniques at any time of the day and in practically any situation.

Now at this point it is extremely important to note that for purposes of simplicity we have been speaking of tension and all of its implications as a "bully," a "villain," as though it were actually an opponent pitted against you. But this is not really the case. The tensions, whatever they may be, *are really a part of you.* As you invite them in and practice your Yoga techniques, you terminate an imaginary split; you end the war you have been fighting with yourself. You tend to become whole again. Great energies which have been tied up are released and you find yourself able to function more and more harmoniously. The essence of the entire procedure is this: *you do not defeat or suppress the tension; you assimilate it!* As this assimilation occurs, not only are you able to regain your natural ability to relax but you can once again grow, mature and develop emotionally as well as in all aspects of your life.

Tension has become such a great source of concern that we are continually confronted with theories and suggestions for relieving tension. It is interesting that a great deal of such advice has to do with using the "mind" to help overcome this problem. We are presented with various methods of auto-suggesting ourselves into states of relaxation. Professional hypnosis is occasionally used for attempting to overcome tension. There have been varying degrees of success with these methods, although it is generally agreed that such results are only temporary. Then, too, we have what is known as "psycho-somatic" therapy: the method of attempting to influence the functioning of the body and the emotions through the mind. This has frequently produced excellent results when administered by a competent authority, and there is undoubtedly great merit in this system, although as a science it is still in its infancy. As a result of the voluminous writings and consideration given to the subject of tension and the means suggested for its relief, a considerable number of people have come to believe that dealing with tensions, as well as with many other disturbances, is a case of what is known as "mind over matter." This is an expression which has become very popular in all levels of society. But the idea of "mind over matter" or "mind over emotions" raises some curious questions. When you think, "I will tell myself to relax," exactly what is happening? Who is the "I" who is telling the "self" to relax? What exactly is the "mind" which is placed "over matter"? Is the mind the thinking process that is carried on in the brain or is it something more? How much do you have to know about the nature of your mind and your physical organism before you can actually use your thoughts to properly influence them? And *where* is this "mind"? Is it encased within the physical organism? Is it in the head? When you order yourself to "relax," who is it that is doing the "ordering" and who is it that is supposed to respond and do the "relaxing"? Is there really such a clear distinction as a mind which can "order," and emotions and a body which can "respond"? And what if it is the mind that is the culprit in the first place? What if it is the *mind* which cannot relax? How then can it be qualified to give orders to itself or to the body or emotions to "relax"? And if it is the mind that must relax, then what or who will give the necessary orders to the mind? Because so many people do believe without question that there is a "mind" and a "body," and that these two are quite distinct one from the other, it is important to consider the theory of Yoga regarding the nature of the mind and the body, since this theory has a direct bearing on the entire problem of achieving true, natural relaxation.

From the Yogic viewpoint the body and the mind (together with the emotions) are so interrelated that they are actually inseparable. The mind is not simply the thinking process relegated to the brain but is the sum total of the intelligence which permeates every atom of the physical and subtle organisms. *Whatever affects the body must influence the mind and vice-versa.* Since the mind is present throughout the body and permeates its every atom, the Yoga techniques which we perform to stretch, strengthen and otherwise improve and develop the body must have a correspondingly profound effect on the mind and the emotions. My experience has proven to me beyond a doubt that there is nothing more effective for achieving a natural quieting, relaxing and stabilizing of the mind and emotions than the simple Yoga body stretches and breathing techniques! The beauty of this method is that you need only try these exercises for several minutes to experience the immediate results. There is no auto-suggestion, no self-hypnosis. You do not have to be "conditioned" to the method. You do not even have to believe or have faith in this theory. All that is necessary is that you correctly and seriously do the physical techniques exactly as described. The results speak for themselves. And working with these techniques is both easy and highly enjoyable so that they are suitable for all persons regardless of the type of tension or disturbance. Even those disturbances of a highly serious nature which are being treated by a psychologist or psychiatrist will respond more readily when the patient is able to effect a receptive state through physical and mental relaxation. In the years to come the practice of the Yoga postures and breathing exercises could become an important aid in psychotherapy.

A word should be included here about that sickness which afflicts so many people and is so enervating—insomnia. Again, with insomnia we have a peculiar paradox. When you cannot sleep you worry about not sleeping because you know you will feel miserable the next day; the more you worry about your insomnia the more acute it becomes and the more impossible it is to sleep. It is probably unnecessary to inform people who are addicted to sleeping pills that this is a most unhealthy habit. The side-effects of these drugs are painfully evident to such people. We will not be concerned about why you may have insomnia; let us see rather what can be done about it. There is a special group of Yoga techniques presented at the end of this chapter for promoting a restful sleep and it is made up primarily of a number of the simple stretching postures. This is because "stretching is nature's tranquilizer" and wherever you are able to stretch, you can relieve tension. Thus stretching in those key areas where tension (tightness, stiffness, cramps) accumulates easily, especially before retiring for the night, can be extremely effective in promoting a restful sleep.

Now going back to what we discussed at the beginning of this chapter, there is a very wonderful thing that happens as you begin to gain the feeling of "letting go" (perhaps we should say "regain," for it is the feeling which you experienced as a youth). The "letting go" results in the ability to relax. At first, the experience of deep relaxation may be confined solely to the time you are actually practicing your Yoga exercises. But gradually, this feeling begins to carry over more and more into your everyday activities. As this happens you often find that the work, chores and tasks which were formerly irritating and tiring lose the power to drain your vital force. When you are truly relaxed you can undertake to accomplish any work which is necessary and do it in a most satisfactory manner by expending a minimum of energy. It is a beautiful thing to watch a person who is truly relaxed and composed perform any activity. Do not confuse relaxation with laziness or inertia. Relaxation gives you access to a much greater supply of energy than you may ever have dreamed possible because energy which was trapped and tied up physically and emotionally is freed. This new source of energy is not "nervous" energy; it is steady and can be controlled and used as needed.

To retain the youth and health of your body, mind and

emotions, there is nothing more important and valuable than to cultivate calmness, tranquility, composure, serenity. With these attributes you radiate dignity, confidence and a quiet power.

Here are the techniques to be emphasized for:

Relaxation—Calmness—Tranquility—Composure—Serenity—Insomnia

Re-read the information on page 162

GENERAL RELAXATION

Chest Expansion	(7)
Cobra	(8)
Neck Movements	(9)
Complete Breath	(10)
Shoulder Stand	(11)
Eye Exercises	(12)
Alternate Nostril Breathing	(14)
Alternate Leg Pull	(17)
Head Stand	(20)

INSOMNIA (For practice before retiring)

Cobra (3 times)	(8)
Neck Movements	(9)
Alternate Nostril Breathing (7 rounds)	(14)

IMMEDIATE RELIEF OF EMOTIONAL DISTURBANCES

Alternate Nostril Breathing (7 rounds)	(14)
Direction of the vital force (Chapter 7)	

3. VITALITY AND ENDURANCE;
Awakening and Conserving Your
Sleeping Energies

YOUTH	*AGE*
Vitality—energy— endurance.	Fatigue—weariness— exhaustion.

In the beginning phases of Yoga practice it may seem that the claim of gaining increased energy and vitality is inconsistent with the slow-motion and passive movements which we employ in the exercises. But this is because we have been conditioned to think of energy as a kind "stimulant" which is derived from such things as fast-motion setting-up exercises, a cold shower, a brisk massage; certain drugs (energizers); "quick energy" foods such as the hi-protein powders and drinks; stimulants such as coffee and refined sugar products. But let us examine these and see if we have not been misled in thinking that they actually provide us with energy. It seems that the confusion lies between natural energy, which the body should always possess and use as needed, and those agents which act as stimulants and shock the nervous system, raise the blood sugar level, make the heart beat more quickly temporarily causing the blood to race and quickening the circulation. These all combine to give the illusion of energy.

To the Yogi, exercising as many people do with the quick 1-2, 1-2 setting-up movements for the purpose of feeling better and gaining energy, is the height of folly. "Why," he asks, "actually work to give away what little energy you may have and consciously place unwelcome stress and strain on your entire physical organism when the whole idea should be to *conserve* and *store* energy?" The cat is a classical example of this conservation of energy. He seems to have the ability to store energy so that it is always available to him as needed. He does no setting-up exercises, but he *does* exercise. How?

Watch him carefully and you will observe that he is continually *stretching*. This is an important clue for us.

The cold shower and the brisk massage can make you feel very good for a short time because of the temporary stimulation but these are the most temporary of devices and certainly could not be considered to have any real ability to increase energy and vitality. I think it is important to mention this here because I have had so much experience with executives who have come to rely entirely upon the massage and use of modern gadgets and devices with the mistaken idea that these things will keep them fit and healthy and add to their vitality.

Next, it is a tragic commentary on our civilization that so many people find it necessary to keep themselves going with so-called "energizers." These are drugs which shock the nervous system and appear to increase energy. The tragedy lies in the fact that such drugs must eventually extract their price and the "addict" (although he is usually surprised to be labeled as such) finds that the energizers become less and less effective and that he needs a larger and larger dosage. Eventually his energy is completely depleted, he suffers from exhaustion which can easily result in various physical illnesses, he grows more anxious and more irritated and even a nervous break-down is not uncommon. The degree of damage is dependent on the natural strength and stamina of the individual. Some can withstand the negative effects for years, but nature always catches up and there must be a time of reckoning. The coffee addict who will consume from 3 to 8 cups per day (a habit which is encouraged throughout our nation by the "coffee break" with conveniently placed machines for the dispensing of coffee) is also well aware of the symptoms of anxiety, irritability, insomnia and other effects, although he may be reluctant to admit to these. The caffeine in coffee provides a momentary stimulation but as this stimulation subsides there is the desire for another cup and then another. You probably know many people who cannot get their eyes open in the morning or remain grouchy and irritable until they have a few cups of coffee. A similar effect is often produced from the refined sugar products such as candy, cakes, cola drinks, etc., a temporary stimulus occurs from the raising of the level of blood sugar but soon this level falls and then more and more sugar is required to raise the level. The implications are obvious: a vicious circle is initiated which is usually broken only when the eventual damage done to the body or the emotions and mind reaches such proportions that the physician will require the patient to discontinue the use of the harmful stimulants.

Finally, in connection with stimulants, I should like to mention briefly what I call the "hi-protein fad." We do not minimize the importance and necessity of protein as nature intended that it be derived from certain foods. But from the Yogic viewpoint we are not in accord with the idea of protein as it is offered to us in crash diets, powders, wafers, mixes and drinks where the body is literally set on fire and burns itself up. In Yoga, we do not want "quick energy." We do not wish to set a straw bonfire which will blaze up and then quickly die out unless we constantly add to the blaze. What we want is *steady* energy, energy which we can conserve and store and then use as necessary. A continual small, controlled flame which does not require the body to work overtime is our objective in the field of energy and vitality.

For the Yoga method of gaining and maintaining the youthful characteristics of energy and vitality we must refer to the four statements which appear on page 11 regarding the nature of the vital force. I suggest that you review these points now. For the practical purposes of this study we can consider the vital force to be synonymous with energy and vitality. Therefore, we can say that there is great energy which lies asleep within you. At this very moment you probably have more energy than you might imagine, but it is buried and it cannot be tapped unless you make a definite effort to do so. Just as the cat retains his energy through stretching, so can we begin to tap and use our reservoir of energy (vital force) through methodical stretching and other careful manipulations of the body. There are particular areas, or "centers," in the body where energy is concentrated and the Yoga exercises which you are now practicing place particular emphasis on these areas; the entire spine, the brain, and many of the organs and glands are such centers. When these centers are stimulated through the natural Yoga movements of the body they release their energy slowly and steadily. The results of having access to this energy will be self-evident and we would venture to state that there is no person who practices according to the plan outlined in this book who will not experience the results of increased energy and vitality.

Regarding foods and their connection with the subject of energy, you will actually be draining your vitality and defeating our objective of gaining steady, controlled energy if you over-indulge in coffee, refined-sugar products, meat products and the various hi-protein formulae. Unless otherwise instructed by your physician, a diet with moderate amounts of meat (organ meats are best, particularly liver), fresh-water fish, whole-milk products, fresh cheeses, whole grains (in breads and cereals), avocados, legumes (dried beans, lentils, peas), and particularly *unroasted* and unsalted nuts such as the cashew, almond, pecan, walnut, Brazil nut and natural nut butters should provide you with an abundance of natural, high-quality protein. It is our opinion that the next several years should see a decline in the current popularity regarding high protein.

Now a more subtle but extremely important aspect of energy should be taken into consideration. If you adhere to the above suggestions regarding foods and seriously follow your Yoga practice plan you will definitely experience an increase in your energy and vitality. It must be pointed out that there are certain ways in which this increased energy may be dissipated or drawn from you without your being aware that this is happening. It seems to be a law of the universe that those people who have an inadequate supply of vital force (which we are now considering as synonymous with energy) are often unconsciously able to draw it from those who have more than they. You probably recall how you have been drawn to certain people who have a type of "magnetic" quality and who seem to radiate vital force and vitality. You draw upon this vitality and come away from contact with this person feeling stimulated, elevated and alive. People who radiate this type of vitality are relatively rare, although you may be fortunate to number one or two such personalities among your acquaintances. By the same token you are probably aware of the many contacts which you make each day that leave you feeling quite negative. That is, when you are in the presence of certain people or groups, your energy is drained and depleted, most of the time without your being aware that this is happening, and you come away tired and numb. As you continue to develop in mind and body through your Yoga practice you will not feel the effects of such a loss of energy; on the contrary, you will act as a generator for many people who will be able to draw much needed energy and vitality from you and you in turn will be continually reimbursed with vital force. It will become a source of great satisfaction for you to transmit your power and energy in a restrained and intelligent manner to others. But in the early phases of your practice, while you are tapping, accumulating and storing energies, it is desirable that you conserve as much of your vital force as possible. An important way of accomplishing this is to attempt to avoid contacts with persons and groups whom you know leave you feeling negative. The slightest analysis on your part will quickly enable you to determine who such people and groups are. Naturally it is not always practical to avoid such contacts and under many circumstances this will be impossible. When such people are members of your own household or when they constitute part of your business relations it is obviously impossible to avoid their company. So we will simply state that "whenever possible" do not risk involving yourself in conditions which you know can drain your energies. You will be surprised at how many negative situations you can eliminate from your daily life with just a little thought and planning. For the time being, if you should find yourself in what appears to be an irritating situation, it is best to assume the most *passive* attitude possible. Of course, that is the advantage which people who intend to embark upon a spiritual life have when they go to a retreat; all external disturbances and unpleasantness can be temporarily eliminated while inner strength and harmony is being developed. But most of us do not have this opportunity and we must effect a transition in the midst of our ordinary everyday life. Even so, it is possible to eliminate a great number of circumstances that lead to bitterness and frustrations and you should take advantage of every opportunity to steer clear of anything which will sap your new-born energies. As your vital force increases, circumstances which were formerly fraught with mental and emotional pitfalls and dangers lose their power to disturb you and you find yourself less and less involved in such situations altogether. This is because as you grow and develop internally so does the external world have a corresponding change. If there is internal harmony you automatically project this into your external world. This is not a metaphysical speculation but a fact which you will experience.

A certain amount of self-observation will also prove valuable in discovering how you may be losing energy needlessly. If several times each day you make it a point to observe the way in which you are moving and holding your body you will find some important clues. You may notice, for example, that you have a continual tendency to hold certain muscles in your legs, abdomen, chest and neck tensed and rigid even when you are doing something which does not require the use of those particular muscles. Many people who perform all of their day's work seated at a desk are physically exhausted at the end of the workday. Poor posture, not taking advantage of a few natural stretching movements during the day and groups of muscles which are almost continually held tensed are responsible for this exhaustion. Such people would benefit greatly by detecting which muscles are involved in this unconscious stress and make repeated attempts to relax these muscles whenever they are found to be needlessly contracted.

Also, you may find that you are unknowingly expending great amounts of energy through so-called "nervous habits." These take the form of incessant foot or hand-tapping, chewing gum, grinding or clenching of teeth, etc. It requires a great expenditure of energy to indulge in a habit such as the chewing of gum. One of my students, a mathematician, once computed the exact amount of energy necessary to chew a stick of gum for several hours. I no longer have these figures but I can assure you that the output of energy was startling! We all know that it is very difficult to overcome any or all of our nervous habits through "will power" or by using that technique already discussed, "mind over matter." As a matter of fact, although I know it would be of very great value to many of my students to cut down or completely stop their smoking (which I classify largely as a nervous habit), I have never yet told a student to "stop smoking." I believe that this is like saying, "You must relax." "Yes, I know I must," answers the student, "but *how?*" We have had great success with overcoming tension of the muscles and terminating nervous habits, including that of smoking, without forcing the issue or having the student make himself feel guilty or inadequate. As with everything in Yoga, this has taken place naturally. When you practice Yoga you will automatically increase your vital force; the vital force works for you in every imaginable way. Increased vital force means increased energy and power for the physical, emotional and mental organisms. These organisms know very well what is in their best interests and if you allow the intelligence and wisdom of the body and mind to operate more freely (which is exactly what happens as you raise your vibrations through the practice of Yoga) you will find yourself increasing those activities which act in a positive manner and automatically decreasing those activities which have a negative effect. Therefore, an *increase* in vital force means a *decrease* in harmful habits. The intelligence of the organism will not allow you to destroy yourself and it will gradually lessen your desires and appetites to indulge in habits which are against the plan of nature. Many Yoga students have stopped smoking for no other reason than the fact that they "just lost the taste for it." In the same manner, the relaxation of muscles and the termination of nervous habits has occurred simply because the tension which made them necessary disappeared. The increase in vitality which has resulted from being able to conserve energy which was formerly being burned up is practically unbelievable. Again, the Yogi is not concerned with whether you believe this to be true, whether it makes sense or whether you have "faith." Simply practice your Yoga techniques exactly as outlined and the results will be the proof.

Endurance is very much tied up with this discussion regarding energy. We are not necessarily referring to the endurance of the athlete in a prolonged sporting event which requires a tremendous physical reserve. We are concerned here with the type of endurance which each of us must have to do our everyday work and to do it with a sense of accomplishment and fulfillment. Endurance is both physical and mental in the sense that not only must you have the necessary physical energy for the required activities but you must also be able to maintain a mental attitude and emotional stability which makes this work important and meaningful. To vast numbers of people, their work is pure drudgery; they go through the movements of their job in a mechanical manner, without interest. They find their duties dull and boring and cannot wait for the day to end. The same is unfortunately true with an alarmingly high percentage of students. Working or studying under such conditions, waiting for the whistle to blow, the bell to ring or the next coffee break, the worker must eventually become highly irritable, nervous, depressed and inefficient. Without realizing it, he is actually frustrated over his inability to be interested in, or to experience a sense of achievement through, his work. At the other end of the scale we have an equally frustrated person. He is the man who wants to be a success in his work but finds endless obstacles arising between himself and his objective. His efforts become more and more frantic but he never really succeeds in overcoming what appears to be "endless obstacles." Why?

Now there is no doubt that many jobs do not require more than a mechanical type of labor, or that many people are engaged in work which seems dull to them because their abilities actually exceed those which their jobs require. It is also true that many jobs appear to present great obstacles so that real success seems to recede further and further beyond the clutching fingers of the person intent upon succeeding. In all of these there is a factor well worthy of our consideration, a possibility which may account for the drudgery or frustration in work. Let us call this the "endurance factor." This endurance factor is best explained by the experience and realization that when a new and abundant influx of energy, as is produced by the stimulation of the vital force, is made available to the organism, there are powerful implications physically, emotionally and mentally. All worldly activity, all work takes on new significance, new importance and often exciting new possibilities. There is a kind of "breakthrough," and one finds that not only does he possess the necessary physical power to do what is necessary without tiring but that there is a corresponding emotional and mental force which now sustains him during his labors and indeed, even encourages him in his work.

It seems that the "let-downs" which are chiefly responsible

for the boredom, drudgery and frustrations vanish as the natural power to "endure" is developed. Understand that here again, this is not a *forced* endurance like that of the Spartan athlete who is committed to run the last mile of the marathon even if he explodes in the attempt, or the Biblical Job-like ability to "endure" afflictions while suffering each moment. We are now speaking of a sustaining power which is so natural that one is not even aware of its action. Then, too, the physical and mental aspects of endurance complement one another in a harmonious duet: as you gain new physical energy to put into your labors, you automatically become more interested in what you are doing; the more interested you become the more you want to see it done correctly and efficiently; the more you are interested in efficiency and devising new ways in which to be efficient, the less you are going to be waiting for the whistle to blow. The increased energy has given you the necessary physical and mental drive for the "breakthrough," which is an escape from the dictatorship of your job. You are no longer tied to your job as a slave. You are the master of your work, regardless of what it is.

It is appropriate to refer here to the greatest book regarding "work" and "action" that is available to man. This guide is the *Bhagavad-Gita,* which constitutes the Yogic viewpoint of all activity. We are told in this ancient book of wisdom that to work is not only a privilege but a great opportunity. All work is of equal importance regardless of its nature and through one's work it is possible to grow and mature, to expand consciousness and develop awareness, to gain harmony and peace and even, eventually, to achieve self-realization. But we are informed that the work must be performed in a particular manner; it cannot be forced but must *flow* from you. You must be so immersed in your work that you *become* your work and lose the ego concept of "I am working." As long as you retain the feeling of "I am working," work will be hard. It is the knowledge, the thought of work, which makes it tedious. When is work not *work?* When it is done simply for its own sake, without one eye continually on the outcome or a desperate concern with what the *Bhagavad-Gita* calls the "fruits of your labor," that is, how much you are going to get out of this job. With this attitude, work is accomplished with a much greater ease and efficiency and the rewards are more than you could have imagined because these rewards are not simply material but spiritual. However, you cannot fake this attitude any more than you can fake the bravado of facing the dragons of tension as already discussed. There has to be an all-consuming interest and inner joy in your labors, and it is necessary to let go of the frantic desire for success. In this way you will always remain free from the grasping tentacles of disappointment and frustration inherent in any work motivated primarily by the greatest possible gain. You are probably thinking, "But how can you have a job and not be deeply concerned with that job? After all, the necessities of life for myself and my family depend on the outcome of my work. How can I not want to beat out the other fellow and try to make the most money from my job? This idea of letting go may be all right if you live in a forest but I live in a highly competitive society," etc. To which the Yogi answers, "Letting go does not imply indifference. You can do whatever you have to do but you can still do it and retain your freedom." The difficulty in further discussion along these lines lies in the fact that the reader may be attempting through his intellect to imagine a state of existence which can only be *experienced!* You cannot accurately *know* a state of consciousness through thinking. You must experience this state. When we tell you that you will feel better if you methodically stretch your body, you may be able to imagine yourself feeling better but if you haven't stretched as advised then imagining is all you *can* do. You can't feel it; you can't experience it. Now, what we are saying here is that this state of freedom and fulfillment as it pertains to work must be experienced. This will be possible through the stimulation of the vital force which results in an extremely profound form of energy, vitality and endurance.

It has also been the experience of a number of students that in gaining the increased vital force, opportunities for work which is more in line with their abilities have gravitated to them. You may make of this what you will but it seems to be a law that the inner harmony which is achieved by the earnest student is reflected in his activities and you will almost always find that one who has seriously practiced Yoga for a period of time is involved in a type of work which is in harmony with his nature. He is not separate from his work; his work is a part of him and he is therefore at peace with both himself and the world.

The physical advantages of gaining energy, vitality and endurance are obvious in our quest for a second youth. But another important and more subtle point which we have attempted to make is this: a person who is bored or is in any way frustrated in his work is definitely going to show the symptoms of age, since irritation, frustration, fatigue and nervousness must take their toll on the organism. So we may now state that the peace and harmony which results from fulfillment through work is an equally important characteristic of youth.

Here are the techniques to be emphasized for:

Vitality—Energy—Endurance

Re-read the information on page 162

Arm and Leg Stretch	(5)
Chest Expansion	(7)
Cobra	(8)
Complete Breath	(10)
Shoulder Stand	(11)
Locust	(15)
Head Stand	(20)

4. BLOOD CIRCULATION;
Using The Life-Fluid to Stay Young

YOUTH	AGE
Proper blood circulation resulting in the health and strength of vital organs and glands.	Inadequate blood circulation with resultant dull complexion, wrinkles; general poor health.

In Yoga we speak about the blood as being the *life-fluid* of the body. We need not become too involved with the reasons for maintaining good blood circulation and making sure that this life-fluid is able to circulate freely throughout the organism to do its work. Everyone is more or less aware that good circulation leads to health and vitality and that poor circulation results in degrees of fatigue and illnesses, of which there can be many. It is not our intention to infringe upon the province of the physician in dealing with problems pertaining to blood circulation which require medical attention. However, there are many people whose over-all health and vitality could be greatly improved just by making a few simple movements daily to promote good circulation.

With certain of the Yoga postures you are probably aware that we are concentrating primarily on improvement of circulation because you can feel what is happening. We are referring specifically to the HEAD and SHOULDER STANDS. When you stand on your head, especially in the early attempts, the reversal in the flow of the blood is obvious and you can feel it pulsating throughout your neck and head. At first the inversions may seem unnatural and sometimes uncomfortable although you can generally feel that there are important benefits which will result. It is very interesting to note (and you may have already found this to be true for yourself) that within a few weeks the discomfort disappears and you feel less and less of an obvious change in the flow of the blood when in the inverted positions. Soon you can remain in these positions for the time suggested without feeling the slightest discomfort; indeed, the inverted postures actually act as agents for relaxation. In the HEAD STAND we are making a direct effort to bring the blood into the head with all of the wonderful benefits which will result. In the SHOULDER STAND we are aiming specifically at the thyroid glands in the neck area. In both of these postures we also want temporarily to bring the blood out of the legs in order to relax them. These effects will be obvious to you because for the most part you can feel very strongly what is happening. But there are other postures acting to improve circulation which are more subtle and their effects may be somewhat difficult to detect. It is valuable to point out a few of these.

The COBRA posture seems to bring an increased blood supply into the kidneys. In the extreme raised position of the COBRA the blood is said to drain from the kidneys and when the trunk is once again lowered the blood flows back into the kidneys, nourishing and in a sense "flushing" them. Among many interesting examples is that of a middle-aged woman who, after practicing the COBRA seriously for several weeks (because she found it beneficial for insomnia) suddenly passed a kidney stone, much to the amazement of her physician, who had not suspected that such a deposit was present. So we definitely know that the COBRA has a very pronounced effect on the kidneys. The LOCUST and the PLOUGH postures bring increased supplies of blood into the heart, the arms and the upper areas of the trunk. The same is true with the backward and forward bends of the CHEST EXPANSION posture. Therefore, a routine incorporating these postures should go far in promoting good circulation in an easy, natural manner without strain. An improvement in circulation can help in normalizing blood pressure, and this possibility should be discussed with your physician. It is my hope that in view of the tremendous amount of therapeutic value which has resulted from Yoga, physicians in all fields of practice will be inclined to take a close look at the Yoga postures and techniques with the possibility of prescribing their use for patients. Technical information regarding the Yoga exercises will soon be available to physicians who are interested.

We should not overlook the COMPLETE BREATH in this discussion. The vital force which we take from the air during the breathing process (and remember that vital force is far more than oxygen) is the agent which nourishes and purifies the life-fluid (blood). It is not enough simply to improve the circulation. We want to be sure that the *quality* of the blood which is being circulated is high. You can purify your blood through frequent practice of the COMPLETE BREATH and by eating foods which contain healthy amounts of the blood-building elements. A list of foods which are rich in these elements is presented in Chapter 7 in the section devoted to "Foods." The COMPLETE BREATH can be done in groups of 25 while walking (coordinate the rhythm of your steps with the counting and movements of the breathing but do not raise your shoulders) and even while driving. As a matter of fact, whenever you can think to do so during the day, take at least a few COMPLETE BREATHS and you will experience an immediate lift.

Many of the symptoms of age respond positively when proper blood circulation is sustained over a period of several months. A few examples should be of interest. Falling hair, which is certainly characteristic of aging, is often checked through the inverted postures, particularly the HEAD STAND. You cannot grow hair once it has fallen out but you can certainly help to check it by bringing the blood into the scalp and nourishing the hair follicles. Dull, lifeless hair regains its sheen and becomes alive once again, and it is fascinating to note that some students have actually had streaks of gray in their hair turn back to the natural color! I cannot promise that this last statement will prove true for you but it is certainly worth a try since you have everything to gain and nothing to lose (that is, except your hair).

Wrinkles, poor complexion and sallow skin, not only in the face but throughout the body, are some of the most obvious and unsightly symptoms of age. We can attribute these symptoms often to a lack of rich, pure blood which is amply supplied to every cell of the body. Many wrinkles are caused by the accumulation of toxins and waste matter in various areas of the body (such as the face) which are not properly eliminated because the blood, whose job it is to carry away toxins, does not properly circulate in these areas. So instead of being carried away by the blood these waste products will crack the skin in order to come out. It should therefore be stressed that the problem of maintaining a smooth, youthful skin and complexion is essentially an *internal* one, and we will discuss this concept again in connection with "Muscle Tone" in the next chapter. But we have seen over and over how a poor, dull, lifeless skin and complexion can change into a radiant and glowing one almost miraculously when a person (1) attempts to ensure proper circulation through the routine of Yoga exercises prescribed for this purpose at the end of this chapter; (2) eliminates from his diet refined-sugar products, white-flour products, coffee, cola drinks, harsh condiments, foods which are rich, fatty and fried, and replaces these with natural, wholesome blood-building foods as will be discussed; (3) maintains the purity and high quality of the blood by promoting good elimination through such techniques as the AB-DOMINAL LIFT.

I should add here that having had many teenagers in my classes, I know that skin eruptions, acne, etc., which are usually taken as "natural" for that stage of life, respond very well to the above program. Nothing could be more *unnatural* than the breaking out of the skin in unsightly eruptions (at any age), and if you will have a teenager follow our exercise and food program earnestly for 1 month there should be a remarkable improvement if not a complete clearing up of the skin. Youngsters respond quickly to the program, adults require a longer period of time, but with both groups the results are more than gratifying.

Think of the blood as the precious life-fluid of your body and know that you can feel and appear only as young as it is rich in quality and properly circulated.

Here are the techniques to be emphasized for:

IMPROVEMENT OF BLOOD CIRCULATION

Re-read the information on page 162

Chest Expansion	(7)
Cobra	(8)
Complete Breath	(10)
Shoulder Stand	(11)
Locust	(15)
Plough	(18)
Head Stand	(20)

5. MUSCLE TONE;
Firmness Without Exertion

YOUTH	*AGE*
Resilience of muscles resulting in firmness, taut skin; strength.	Loss of muscle tone resulting in sagging, flabbiness; weakness.

When you lose muscle tone, the skin which these muscles are supporting must sag. It's as simple as this: poor muscle tone—flabbiness and skin which withers and sags; good muscle tone—firm body and taut skin. Here again the key to youth is *stretching*. Conscientious stretching firms and develops muscles in accordance with their natural potential. I should like to caution all male readers to consider very carefully before deciding to overdevelop muscles through weight-lifting and the various gadgets and devices which are designed for such overdevelopment. The great stress and strain placed on the muscles, organs and glands through gadgets which require strenuous pushing, pulling and lifting can very definitely prove harmful in many ways. And in addition, as we have already mentioned, unless this strenuous procedure is continued once the muscles have been overdeveloped, this muscle will turn into fat and then the "muscle man" is in real trouble. We have exactly this situation with numerous professional athletes. Overdevelopment of the body is directly opposed to the Yoga theory of natural development with the least possible exertion. People who are active in various sports may overdevelop to some extent certain groups of muscles but, in general, this is not harmful if not overdone.

From the health standpoint, the maintenance of muscle tone is absolutely indispensable. For example, when the resilience is lost in the abdominal muscles, many of the organs and glands which are supported by that abdominal wall will begin to drop. These organs will then tend to push and press other organs and the implications are obvious. From the appearance standpoint, a most unsightly symptom of aging occurs when the abdomen begins to fall into the groin area. We can avoid and in many cases help to correct this occurrence through the SHOULDER and HEAD STANDS and the ABDOMINAL LIFT. In the inverted positions the organs and glands of the viscera, which may be out of position tend to revert to their natural position which is high in the viscera. The abdomen will be relieved of the pressure due to the continual downward pull of gravity in the usual standing and sitting positions and gravity now works for us by pulling the abdomen in the opposite direction. The slow raising and lowering of the legs in the SHOULDER STAND exercise will also act to strengthen the abdominal muscles. In the ABDOMINAL CONTRAC-

TION and LIFT movements we make a very concentrated effort to raise the abdomen and greatly strengthen the abdominal muscles as well as to return organs which may have been pushed out of place to their natural position. The value of the ABDOMINAL LIFT becomes extremely significant when you realize that there is practically no activity during everyday life which makes us use and exercise these vital muscles!

The thighs and calves can be firmed and the flabbiness reduced through a number of the exercises. The LEG PULLS, the BACKWARD BEND, the KNEE and THIGH STRETCH, the LOCUST, the BOW and the PLOUGH are a most dynamic routine of movements for firming, developing and putting youthful spring back into your legs. Each of these exercises works out the legs and thighs in a slightly different manner and every muscle is gently stretched and strengthened. The thoroughness of these postures can only be appreciated when you are actually concentrating on the movements and attempt to *feel* what is happening. Notice how the LEG PULLS stretch and firm the *back* of the thighs and calves; how the BACKWARD BEND works on the *front* part of the thighs; how the KNEE and THIGH STRETCH firms the *inside* of the thighs; how the TOE TWIST, ARM and LEG STRETCH, LOCUST, BOW and PLOUGH strengthen and streamline the legs.

The LOCUST posture brings into play seldom-exercised muscles in the legs and groin. You realize how weak these important muscles have grown when you first attempt the LOCUST as described in this book. But there is more to the LOCUST than the development of the leg and groin muscles. According to the yogis, the LOCUST has a most stimulating and strengthening effect on the reproductive organs and glands. The same is true, to a lesser degree, of the PLOUGH posture. Therefore, emphasis on a combination of the LOCUST and PLOUGH can often aid in virility in the male, and, in the female, by strengthening the position of the organs and glands, can help to prevent or possibly correct certain disorders of the womb and uterus, which may be out of position.

For reducing flabbiness in the hips and strengthening the lower back, the BOW posture should be emphasized. After you have learned to do the BOW well, you should attempt the following variation: in the extreme position, with your trunk and knees raised from the floor, begin a gentle rocking motion on the groin and abdomen. This must be a very slow and controlled movement. In the forward movement of the roll you will move onto the abdomen; in the backward movement you will roll onto the groin but you remain holding your ankles with your trunk raised throughout these movements. Repeat the rocking motion from 5 to 10 times.

Flabbiness and loss of muscle tone in the upper arms is a definite sign of aging and is a common complaint even among young women. Naturally, when the muscles in this area lose their tone the skin will give the effect of age because it grows flabby and sags. There are four exercises among those in this book which can be highly recommended for the firming of the upper arms. These are: the CHEST EXPANSION (the stretching and firming as the arms are held high throughout the backward and forward bends); the ARM and LEG STRETCH (bringing the upraised arm backward); the LOCUST (pushing down hard with the fists while raising the legs); the HEAD STAND (the weight of the entire body supported by the head and arms). As you are able to firm your upper arms through the practice of these techniques you will find that excess weight in this area can be automatically reduced and redistributed as necessary.

The muscle tone in the neck and face can be greatly promoted simply by bringing the blood into these areas through the inverted postures already described in the chapter on "Blood Circulation." Let me repeat again that the problem of a firm and taut skin in the neck and face areas is essentially an *internal* one. Bringing the blood into the face and stretching the muscles of the neck and face daily will do more to prevent the skin in the neck and face from sagging than all the machines, massages, creams, ointments and other agents which you can use. The NECK MOVEMENTS are good for improving muscle tone. There is another excellent Yoga exercise which you can practice a few times before retiring. This technique is equally valuable for men and women and is known as the LION posture. The movements consist of widening the eyes, opening the mouth wide and extending the tongue out as far as is possible. The object is to feel all of the muscles in the face and neck stretching and to hold the position with the eyes wide and the tongue extended way out for approximately 30 seconds. This movement can be done 5 times. If you are worried about looking peculiar and do the posture timidly you will not reap the benefits which are possible.

Remember that it is the muscles which support the skin and you cannot truly strengthen these muscles with machines, gadgets or by the external applications of creams; firming comes through stretching and only *you* can stretch and tone your muscles through correct exercise.

Here are the techniques to be emphasized for:

MUSCLE TONE

Re-read the information on page 162

LEGS and THIGHS

Preliminary Leg Pull	(1)
Knee and Thigh Stretch	(2)
Backward Bend	(3)
Toe Twist	(4)
Arm and Leg Stretch	(5)
Locust	(15)
Bow	(16)
Alternate Leg Pull	(17)
Plough	(18)
Complete Leg Pull	(19)

ABDOMEN

Abdominal Lift	(13)
Shoulder Stand	
(raising and lowering of legs)	(11)

ARMS

Arm and Leg Stretch	(5)
Chest Expansion	(7)
Locust	(15)
Head Stand	(20)

NECK and FACE

Neck Movements	(9)
Shoulder Stand	(11)
Head Stand	(20)
Lion (Chapter 5)	

6. NORMALIZING WEIGHT; Letting Nature Take Over

YOUTH	*AGE*
Normal weight (in accordance with bone structure) and ability to control and distribute weight.	Obesity; inability to control and maintain correct weight.

If you are overweight you do not need to be given reasons why you *must* reduce excess pounds. You are very well aware of the strain on your heart, the stress on your internal organs, the heaviness in body and mind and the distortion in appearance. But the problem almost always is that it seems to be such a terrible chore, requiring much unpleasant work and sacrifice to lose those life-shortening pounds. In Yoga, however, we have a unique and wonderfully natural approach to this problem. We cater to nature and allow the wisdom of the body to take over the work.

You will remember that it is not the *amount* of movement which a person undertakes which will eventually act to normalize and correctly distribute his or her weight. It is the *type* of movement. We cannot overemphasize this point because there are so many Americans who at this very moment are attempting to "work off" their extra pounds by subjecting themselves to quick, forceful, strenuous movements which make their pulses race, their hearts pound and leave them exhausted. These strenuous movements are probably doing more harm than good in the majority of cases and can result in a weakening of the heart muscles. This type of quick, strenuous movement seems especially useless since it never results in more than a most temporary reduction of extra pounds. These pounds will quickly return if the exercises are discontinued for even a short period of time. It is my opinion that the same is true in using the various machines, apparatus and devices which are supposed to "trim you and firm you." They are also a most temporary means of coping with the problem. The same is true with steam rooms, which many people prize so highly and unfortunately use as a substitute for methodical exercise. Continual heat places a definite strain on the internal organs and you will almost always notice your heart beating more quickly in the steam bath.

"Are you saying that with the Yoga exercises you can normalize and control weight permanently, and that if you stop practicing Yoga the weight will not return?" This is the question asked by nearly everyone to whom I speak. My answer, from a great deal of experience, is "Yes" to the first part of the question and "No" to the second part. That is, if you will perform your "Complete Plan of Practice" and emphasize the techniques listed at the end of this chapter, and if you will follow a sensible diet, you can definitely normalize and thereafter control your weight permanently. The wonderful part of these weight-control movements is that they are performed, as you already know, without strain to the body and with very little real effort. The Yoga postures are designed to stimulate and promote the correct functioning of the important organs and glands of the body which are weight factors and which receive so little conscious attention in the usual systems of calisthenics, in sports and in the use of machines and apparatus. Specifically, you will be working on the thyroid glands; you will be improving blood circulation; you will be breathing in a way designed to help burn excess fat; you will be firming and strengthening many areas of your body, and you will find that when these areas become firm, weight can be much more easily removed.

As to the weight returning if you stop practicing Yoga, I do not hesitate to state that you will never stop practicing Yoga. Yoga is not work; it is fun and it is enjoyable. Once learning and practicing Yoga, even for a short time, you will find that you will never want to discontinue the exercises. Because the Yoga exercises produce a slow and steady improvement and sense of well-being you may not realize how elevated and "alive" you have become until you stop practicing for a few days. Then you may feel a vague let-down, which is an indication that the vital force which you have awakened is no longer being properly stimulated. Your body will then literally compel you to do your Yoga exercises because it knows intuitively that this is what is required in order to once again experience the feeling of functioning at your best. This is what we mean when we say that "nature takes over." You need never be concerned about what happens if you stop practicing Yoga because there is every indication that your body will never allow you to go for long without doing these enjoyable, wonderful exercises—not as a chore but as one of the most stimulating activities of your day.

It is important to note in connection with weight reduction

that the general structure of the body must be considered. For example, people who have a large bone structure should not attempt to reduce their weight beyond what is correct for this structure. Your physician can inform you regarding your proper weight. If your weight is correctly proportioned, your muscles and skin taut and firm, your posture and carriage erect and you are "thinking gracefully" by moving with poise and balance, you can have a large bone structure and never appear overweight; on the contrary, you will reveal yourself as confident, vital and harmonious, as was nature's intention. The point here is, especially for our female readers: never reduce beyond the safe point, attempting to look like the models in the magazines or indiscriminately following the charts on the public scales, since you may find that your health suffers. Your physician should be consulted if you are in doubt as to your correct weight.

Now it would be misleading in this discussion to imply that insufficient and incorrect exercising is the sole factor in the problem of weight normalization and control. *Your diet plays an equally important role.* The subject of sensible and nutritious eating from the Yogic standpoint is outlined in Chapter 7. But I think that it is important as well as extremely interesting to note here the Yogi's view on several matters of dieting for weight control. We would like to call your attention once again to what was mentioned in Chapter 3, the current hi-protein fad. Unless your physician has specifically placed you on such a diet, the Yogi is not in accord with the idea of setting the body on fire and attempting to have it burn itself up. This increased metabolic activity is not conducive to the quiet, relaxed and passive state of mind and body which we wish to attain in Yoga. This state of agitation results when high protein is the mainstay of a diet in which large amounts of meats, poultry, fish and eggs are used in each meal. Such things as appetite "killers," designed to reduce the normal desire for nourishment, a voluntary coffee and cigarette diet, the synthetic products which are taken in liquid form in the place of food, the 30-day miracle "crash" diet which appears in the Sunday supplements, are all in conflict with our concept of natural weight reduction and control. If you will undertake the regular practice of Yoga, performing the exercises daily exactly according to the instructions, and if you will eat a sensible, wholesome, nourishing diet, you will find that your weight will be progressively normalized and will remain at that point which is correct for you. Do not expect a sudden, magical transformation. This is not a "crash" program, which generally results in more harm than benefit. Nature cannot be fooled, tricked or compromised. If it has taken you several years or longer to gain excess weight, you must be sensible and allow nature to progress methodically with her gradual plan. The reward for adhering to nature's method is the permanent control of weight. Surely this is the most intelligent procedure for us to follow.

Although we have so far dealt primarily with the *loss* of weight, those readers who wish to *gain* weight will find that the procedure is practically the same! First you should make sure that you *are* definitely underweight by consulting your physician. If your bone structure is small you do not want to add *excess* weight. You can fill out your frame by making your muscles firm and taut, by methodical stretching to gain flexibility and by learning to move with grace and poise. Again, to attempt to make yourself appear like the muscle men in the magazine advertisements through such devices as the lifting of weights and resorting to the gadgets, apparatus and other so-called "body building techniques" can place a definite strain on your body. If you are truly underweight you may have one or more problems. You may have the problem of assimilation, i.e., no matter how much you eat you do not gain weight because your body is not properly assimilating the food. This can be due to nervousness, which in turn may be attributed to an emotional problem. If this is true, then learning to relax can have a very positive effect on your gaining weight. There are other factors involved but rather than go into these in further detail, let us simply state that if your body requires more weight, the practice of your Yoga exercises coupled with a sensible diet is the very best natural procedure you can undertake for any and all weight problems. Of course, extreme or serious cases involving glandular disorders and emotional problems should always be dealt with by the proper authorities. We should like to note in conclusion that those people who consider themselves "thin" should be aware that it is the Yogi's belief that it is far better to be a few pounds underweight than overweight. You will feel light, you will be clear and alert in your mind and you will probably live longer, as statistics have proven. How many illnesses and deaths could probably be prevented if only we Americans were not quite so "well nourished." The term "well nourished" is, of course, a misnomer, since many Americans are literally starving; although they fill their stomachs very amply three or more times each day, their diets are woefully lacking in the real elements of nutrition.

Now let us see which of the Yoga exercises we can emphasize for weight problems.

Here are the techniques to be emphasized for:

Weight—Normalization—Redistribution—Control

Re-read the information on page 161

REDUCED IN WAIST AND HIPS

Toe Twist	(4)
Abdominal Lift	(13)
Plough	(18)

REDUCED IN BUTTOCKS, THIGHS and LEGS

Backward Bend	(3)
Cobra	(8)
Locust	(15)
Bow	(16)
Plough	(18)

REDUCED IN ARMS

Arm and Leg Stretch	(5)
Chest Expansion	(7)
Locust	(16)

OVER-ALL REDUCTION

Complete Breath	(10)
Shoulder Stand	(11)

OVER-ALL GAINING

Chest Expansion	(7)
Complete Breath	(10)
Shoulder Stand	(11)
Locust	(15)
Head Stand	(20)

7. REGENERATION;
Making the Most of the Elements Which Rebuild

YOUTH	*AGE*
Quick replacement of vital elements continually used by body and brain.	Slowness or loss of ability to replace these vital elements.

An army which has strong reserves and can call up immediate replacements as needed has a very strong advantage over one which must rely solely on its first line of defense and must attempt to regroup whenever there is a breakthrough by the enemy. To successfully wage the battle against age requires just such reserves. If you can always call upon immediate replacements (the vital force in its various manifestations) whenever there is a *deterioration* you will hold the line against the forces of age and will automatically counterattack through *regeneration*. Let us see exactly how it is possible to make certain that we have the necessary reserves.

We have so far been concerned with two sources of the vital force. The first source is the unlocking of the vital force which is *within* the organism as outlined on page 11. Secondly, there are the elements of nature outside of the organism from which the vital force is extracted and used, and we have discussed the foremost of these elements with regard to *air* and how it is used in Complete Breath and Alternate Nostril Breathing. There are other important elements which supply the vital force, and we should learn how to make the most of these from the Yogic viewpoint.

In addition to *air*, the elements involved are *sun, sleep, water* and *food*.

SUN—The sun is a great source of vital force, and life as we know it would probably be impossible without solar energy. However, the student of Yoga should be cautious in the manner in which he accumulates this solar energy. For example, the sun-bath is desirable if taken in moderation, but when one "bakes" himself because he has heard somewhere that the more sun the better, or attempts to get tanned as quickly as possible so that he looks healthy, he is the victim of an erroneous belief and will eventually lose far more vital force than is gained! The direct rays of the sun should be avoided whenever possible during sun-bathing (and this is especially true during the summer months), since they are highly enervating and will drain your energies. The best time for the Yoga student to take the sun is when the rays are somewhat indirect, and this would be approximately before 11 AM and after 2 PM. There may be some variations according to time of the year and geographical location. Do not shower immediately after sunning. Allow the skin an hour to absorb the rays. If you work in the sun, wear a hat to cover your head. If you are on vacation, never attempt to get a tan in one or two days, for you will deplete your vital force and probably suffer in other ways. A mild sun lotion is desirable, especially one which is made from natural elements, without too many chemicals. Such products can generally be purchased from or ordered through a health-food store. For people who live in areas where the winters do not permit exposing themselves to the sun, it is advisable to use a sun lamp for several minutes once or twice a week. It is an excellent idea to practice your Yoga exercises, whenever possible, out-of-doors, and if you can do this while taking the indirect rays of the sun you will feel wonderfully invigorated. An ideal situation would be to practice the exercises first thing in the morning, outdoors, facing the rising sun. This is the method followed by the serious *Hatha* Yogi, who practices in India. Yogis can be seen practicing in this fashion as the sun rises along the banks of the Ganges. The hour of sunset is another ideal time to practice, especially breathing and meditation (which will be explained in Chapter 8), since this is a time of day in which environment is theoretically quiet and the body and mind can be brought into harmony with this peace of the external world. At any rate, do what is most practical for you, but if you ever have the opportunity to practice as suggested above, do not fail to take advantage of it.

SLEEP—Science cannot as yet satisfactorily explain what happens during sleep. However, it is clear that a powerful regeneration takes place, and if a person is prevented from sleeping for a period of time there are severe repercussions physically, emotionally and mentally. Students often ask, "How much sleep is necessary?" There is no definite answer to this question since this is a highly individual matter. Some students do well with 6 or 7 hours. Others cannot function at their best unless they have 8 to 10 hours. You must learn for yourself what the proper number of hours is and make certain that you get in these hours each night. There is nothing which can so quickly lower resistance and break down your reserves as a lack of the correct number of sleeping hours. If you feel exhausted and irritable on a given day, check back and see if you have had adequate sleep the previous night (or you might have missed proper sleep for several nights). As Yogis, we cannot afford this obvious violation of nature's law for the regeneration of the vital force. It may be also, as we have already indicated, that although you retire at an hour which should give you enough sleep, you cannot sleep restfully and you toss and turn so that a number of hours are lost. Perhaps you have too many things racing through your mind and you cannot sleep at all! If this is the case, practice the routine of exercises as advised under "Insomnia" at the end of this chapter. Remember not to eat for at least two hours before retiring. Another question often asked is, "Should you sleep on your side, your back or your abdomen?" Although classic Yogic literature advises sleeping on the right side I have never found any noticeable benefit from one position rather than another. It is beneficial, however, to sleep on a surface (mattress) which offers good resistance and is not too soft, as "sinking into" a mattress can cause stiffness, aches and pains in the back. The more flat the surface the better, and your head should not be raised so high that the blood drains from the upper extremities. Many of my students have tried sleeping without a pillow for several weeks and once they grow accustomed to it they find that they have more energy and clarity upon awakening because of improved circulation. You might experiment with this and see how it affects you. It is interesting to note in passing that during sleep the Yogi will lie so that his head is toward the north and his legs toward the south. He feels that this polarity is in harmony with that of the earth and has a certain "magnetizing" effect. When your senses and perception become refined through the practice of Yoga you may be able to feel that this north-south position increases the regenerating effect of sleep. If it does not present a physical problem you should attempt to sleep with your head toward the north and your feet toward the south.

AIR, WATER—There are a number of important facts regarding the vital elements of air and water worthy of note here. The common denominator for both is *purity*. It is not always possible to exist in an environment where the air is pure, especially if one must work in a large city or live in a heavily populated or industrial area. Exhaust fumes, factory smoke and smog present definite hazards. There is not much that the average person can do about these situations. Air-purifiers, filters, machines that produce "negative ions" are probably helpful to a degree. Whenever possible the student of Yoga should retreat to an area (if only for a few hours) where the air is pure and cleanse and revitalize his blood with plenty of deep and COMPLETE BREATHS. This will prove valuable if done even once a week. Throughout the world it has been realized since time immemorial by civilizations and organizations dedicated to a spiritual life that an environment where the air is charged with *prana* (vital force) was the most satisfactory. Such an environment is located near a body of water or at high altitudes. The latter is most desirable. It is not a coincidence that so many religious retreats and spiritual centers are located in mountains, often at extremely high altitudes. Rarified air is permeated with vital force and you are well aware of the sense of exhilaration which you feel when you are in the mountains. Increased vital force is the reason. The proximity of a large body of water will also impart the sense of well-being, although to a lesser extent. It is of real value to the Yoga student to be in either of these environments whenever possible. Such an environment plays an important role in revitalization and will help build strong reserves. One of the finest activities that it is possible for you to undertake is to find a retreat at a high altitude and spend some time each year in quiet study, in Yoga practice, reflecting on the aspects of nature and meditation. For the person who is dedicated to growth and maturity the retreat is an absolute must. *Awareness* is developed when one is quiet and listens to the silence, or better still, *feels* the silence and allows himself to be instructed through its wisdom.

One can live for many days and even weeks without food. But he cannot live for long without water. The vital force in water is more necessary than food to sustain life. For the student of Yoga the rule regarding water is simple: he will make certain that his drinking water is pure, i.e., that it contains no chemicals. There are as many authorities who strongly oppose the addition of chemicals to the water supplies of the various cities as there are those who support it. I personally do not believe that these chemicals are desirable for the Yoga student simply because I feel that through them the vital force in water is somehow decreased or destroyed. I can offer no scientific proof to substantiate this feeling because to begin with, we are dealing with a highly subtle element in the vital force. I simply do not believe that an element as highly important as water should be tampered with except in cases of emergency. It seems that the strongest argument advanced in favor of the addition of fluorine to the water supply is that it helps to prevent tooth decay. But the real cause of tooth decay is the improper care of the teeth and the eating of foods which promote decay. Decay can be reduced if the food suggestions of this chapter are followed closely. It is our belief that the best water for drinking purposes is obtained from a spring or from mountain streams. For the average city-dweller the best supply of drinking water is obtained through bottled spring water (pure, nothing added), which can be purchased inexpensively in quart or gallon bottles and is ordinarily delivered to a residence by the water companies. Drink only when you are thirsty unless otherwise advised by your physician. There is no such thing as a required amount of water each day. Those people who believe it is necessary to drink a certain number of glasses of water each day to wash out their systems are placing an unnecessary strain on their kidneys. Your body will tell you when it requires water. Here again we learn to trust the wisdom of our own organism, which is completely unique and individual and will instruct us in its exact needs as we learn to listen to and trust it.

FOOD—The last element of the vital force which necessitates our serious consideration is that of food. The student of Yoga who has been practicing for even a relatively short period of time seems to become very much aware that what he eats has a tremendous effect on the way he feels, much more so than before he began his study. He senses that after some meals he feels alive and well and others leave him with a heavy, lethargic, dull feeling. He begins to wonder why this is true and is usually anxious to undertake an investigation. I can safely state that one of the most often-asked questions in this entire study is: "What does the Yogi eat?" This is a difficult question to answer. If we have in mind the Yogi in India then we have to speak about a diet which is for the most part impractical for us to consider simply because of the type of foods involved and their method of preparation. The fact is that it is not so much a question of *what* the Yogi eats as "*why* does he eat at all?" The answer is: "He eats for vital force." If you have been or will be seriously practicing your Yoga techniques and following the other suggestions given to you in this book then you can consider yourself to be a Yogi, a novice (*chela*), perhaps, but a practicing Yogi nonetheless. Therefore, you too must now begin to think about eating not simply to satiate your taste buds or fill up your stomach but for vital force. Foods can give you great reserves of vital force, help regenerate your organism and return to you the characteristics of youth, or they can sap your vital force and add to the symptoms of age. The choice is up to you.

Rather than speak in terms of exact foods, menus, diets, calories, let us think in terms of how we should *feel* from the foods which we eat. Foods should leave us feeling light, energized, revitalized, not heavy and dull. For this feeling of lightness in body and clarity of mind it is necessary to eat foods which are truly nourishing, not those which give the illusion of nourishment. This is an important distinction because simply filling up the stomach can drain more vitality than it adds. Most Americans consider themselves and the population in general to be extremely well nourished but I doubt seriously that this is actually the case. We have plenty to eat but the incredible amount of illness and disease among our population may very possibly be largely attributed to widespread starvation, a starvation for the real elements of nourishment, which are either lacking or present in minimal quantities in the average diet. There are as many conflicting theories regarding the type of nourishment that should be gained from menus and diets as there are people who compile them. Many students who have become involved in a study of nutrition have found the difference of opinions and the resulting confusion to be so overwhelming that they have given up in disgust. It has been my experience that if the student acquaints himself with certain *guiding principles* of nutrition which can be stated in very simple and concise terms, these principles will automatically direct him to the foods which really contain life, or vital force. He can then select and combine these foods intelligently according to *his own particular needs and desires.* Here are the 5 principles:

1. All edible natural foods, i.e., foods which grow and certain animal (milk) products are high in vital force.

2. As natural foods are tampered with they will lose their vital force, proportionately. The term "tampering" refers to refining, canning, preserving, aging, fumigating and cooking or preparing in a manner which renders foods lifeless and indigestible.

3. Foods which contain stimulants should be very moderately consumed by the student of Yoga. Refined-sugar and flour products, coffee, alcoholic beverages and an overabundance of high protein preparations will deplete the vital force.

4. Meat, fish and poultry should be consumed moderately by the student of Yoga.

5. Foods at any one meal should be combined discriminately. A great deal of indigestion, heartburn, gas and other disturbances are caused from mixing foods which simply do not combine.

Before we go into some detail regarding each of these 5 principles, here is a list of what can be regarded as natural foods, high in vital force.

INDEX OF FOODS

SUGARS
Sweet fresh fruits
Molasses
Honey (uncooked, unbleached)
Raw sugar
Beet sugar
Cane sugar (the cane stalks)
Carob (St. John's bread)
Dried fruits: dates, figs, prunes, raisins, apricots, peaches, etc.

STARCHES
Bananas
Brown rice
Potatoes (baked, boiled)
Whole grain breads, crackers
Pumpkin
Barley
Rye

MINERALS (this list includes most fruits and vegetables)
Apples, apricots, artichokes, beets, blueberries, broccoli, brussels sprouts, cabbage, cauliflower, carrots, celery, cherries, cranberries, cucumbers, dandelion, eggplant, endive, garlic, grapes, grapefruit, green peas, green peppers, kale, leeks, lemons, limes, lettuce, melons, mustard greens, oranges, parsley, parsnips, peaches, pears, pineapples, plums, pomegranates, prunes, radishes, raspberries, spinach, rhubarb, strawberries, string beans, squash, tangerines, tomatoes, turnips, watercress.

INDEX OF FOODS (con't)

PROTEINS

Avocados

Legumes (beans, peas, lentils, soy beans and soy bean products)

Nuts (*unroasted and unsalted;* almonds, cashews, pecans, walnuts, Brazil nuts; not peanuts)

Coconuts (and coconut milk)

Nut butter (almond, cashew; not peanut)

Meat (organ meat preferred, particularly beef liver, kidneys, brains)

Poultry (very moderately)

Fish (moderately)

See also "Dairy Foods"

DAIRY FOODS (These are also fats and proteins)

Goat milk

Certified raw milk

Non-fat milk

Yogurt (and all sour milk products)

Cottage cheese (uncreamed)

Farmer cheese

Ricotta cheese (an Italian cheese)

Butter (made from whole milk)

(Buttermilk and sour cream not suggested)

GRAINS

All *whole grain* products (no refined flour products)

CONDIMENTS

All edible herbs

Vegetable salt

OILS (These are also fats)

Saflower oil

Sesame seed oil

Pure olive oil

(Use for cooking and dressings)

BEVERAGES

All fresh fruit and vegetable juices

Vegetable broths

Herb teas

Cereal beverages (coffee substitutes)

This is a general list of natural foods and their products which are high in vital force from the standpoint of our Yoga study. There are other natural foods and their products which certainly can be added to this list according to your own knowledge and desires. But this index will serve as a general indication of what we have in mind and whenever possible, select foods from this list and avoid foods which have been preserved, canned, aged, cooked or otherwise prepared in a manner which seems to conflict with our "natural" concept, for these processes destroy the vital force and have a negative effect on the organism. Preparation of foods should always be in as simple and natural a form as possible. Whenever digestion permits, vegetables should be heated only until they are tenderized. When preparing, cut your vegetables as little as possible as they lose vital force when exposed to oxygen. Whenever possible eat the skin (or at least the inside of the skin) of all fruits and vegetables. Baking and broiling are good methods of cooking but always avoid overcooking as excess heat reduces the vital force. Never fry foods or cook with any substance which produces grease. Many vegetables can and should be eaten raw with a dressing composed of natural oils, lemon juice or other natural preparations available in health-food stores. All vegetable juices (obtained through a vegetable-juice extractor or purchased fresh from the health-food store and certain markets) are excellent and very high in minerals. The same is true for the water in which the vegetables are cooked. Never throw this water away. It should be saved and used as a base for broths and soups. All vegetables from the above list can be combined at a given meal.

Practically all fruits can and should be eaten raw without the addition of sugar. Dried fruits (prunes, figs, etc.) can be soaked overnight in water for easier digestion. All fresh fruit juices are excellent but remember to eat oranges and grapefruits as well as drink the citrus juices. It is important to note that to the Yogi, fruits are fine for cleansing purposes and many students will eat only fruits and their juices one or two days each week for reducing and cleansing. It is not desirable to mix more than a few fruits at any one meal and citrus fruits should never be mixed with dried fruits (oranges with prunes or dates, etc.).

Fresh fruits and vegetables are the most desirable whenever they can be obtained. Frozen fruits and vegetables are the next choice. From our viewpoint, canned or bottled fruits, vegetables and their juices are low in vital force.

The effects of foods which contain stimulants have been discussed in Chapter 3. Regarding alcoholic beverages, an occasional drink will not impede your Yoga practice. A light wine is probably the least harmful of the alcoholic drinks. You need not force yourself to stop drinking. If your body becomes cleansed and your vital force is more active you will automatically lose your desire for alcohol, as was explained in connection with smoking. Alcohol no longer gives you the illusion of a lift or exhilaration. You are able to perceive that in reality alcohol dulls your *natural* sense of exhilaration and produces a very distorted and negative effect on your organism physically, emotionally and mentally.

The subject of meat, fish and poultry is a delicate one. It is extremely difficult in our society to give up eating animal flesh and its by-products even if one truly wishes to do so. Meat and meat products are so much a part of all meals everywhere that you have to be extremely determined and impervious to the scoffing of friends and relatives who will tell you that you are a food 'faddist' or a 'crackpot.' But let us state the case against the eating of meat from the Yogic viewpoint and you can then decide how far you may wish to follow along this line of thinking. The simple fact is that meat will make you feel heavy in body and mind. After your big steak dinner you know that you must rest for a considerable period of time before you can again function normally. Your body is more or less immobile and your mind is dulled. This is because the body requires rest and time to cope with the impact which meat makes upon it. The Yogi feels that a great strain is placed upon the entire digestive system through the continued eating of meat and that the nourishment which one is supposed to derive from meat products is highly overrated. It is our belief that protein of a superior type can be obtained from the other foods listed in the "Index of Foods" under "Proteins" without the heaviness and stress experienced from meat. Our objective in Yoga is to remain light and alert at all times and it cannot be denied that meat produces the exact opposite effect. We are therefore defeating our purpose when we eat any food which seems to deplete our vital force.

The second argument against meat is more subtle and profound. *Meat inhibits the activation of the vital force and the resulting elevation of mind and spirit.* To test this theory you can try a most revealing experiment. As soon as is practical and convenient, set aside a period of 30 days during which you will eat no meat, fish or poultry whatsoever. During this 30-day period you will substitute other proteins as listed in the place of meats so that you will not experience a feeling of hunger (which is a false hunger in most cases) or not lose body weight. (Of course, you *can* lose weight if you wish during this period by eating very little protein.) During this 30-day period you will, unknowingly, become very light in body, keen in sense perception and alert in mind. Since this happens gradually over the month, you cannot appreciate how much of a change has taken place until, at the end of this 30-day period you have yourself a good meat dinner with all of the usual trimmings. The intense let-down and heaviness that occurs physically and mentally after this meal is so revealing that it has often caused a student to decrease greatly and sometimes discontinue altogether his consumption of meat. He realizes how much of his energy and vital force has been continually drained by eating meats. This is a very worth-while experiment and you should try it as soon as possible because one such experiment is worth a great deal of argument, debate and speculation. If one must eat meats, the best meats from the standpoint of this study are organ meats, particularly liver (beef), kidneys, brains. These should be broiled and rare. Poultry cannot in any way be considered superior to meat. Fish is possibly the least harmful of the animal products, especially those fish which feed on sea vegetables rather than other fish. We have already indicated in the "Index of Foods" that certain animal by-products such as milk, cheese and butter are satisfactory, especially those made from goat's milk or raw certified milk (whole milk which has not been pasteurized and homogenized). For those desiring to lose weight, a non-fat milk and dairy products which are low in fat content should be used. A word about eggs: eggs are not as important or necessary as many people seem to think, and there are many proteins, we believe, that are better foods than eggs. If eaten several times a week (especially boiled) they will probably not prove harmful, but it is certainly not advisable that they be made the main breakfast food each day.

Try not to mix too many foods at any one meal. Mark Twain once remarked, "I never worry about what I eat. I just put the foods in my stomach and let them fight it out." We laugh when we read that statement but when we experience the sensation of the "fight" going on within our digestive system it is not very funny. Indiscriminate combinations of foods make digestion very difficult and will produce gas, bloating and other discomforts. Also, the value of foods that may have vital force will be seriously reduced or destroyed. A few examples of categories of foods which should *not* be combined are: fruits with vegetables; fats with starches; fats with proteins. The best rule to follow always is to keep your foods as simple and natural as possible, combining them intelligently and attempting to observe the reactions which they have on you. It cannot be sufficiently emphasized that each person is different in his reactions to foods and their combinations and he must discover for himself the best program to pursue. Therein lies the fallacy of presenting reducing, gaining, cleansing and other type of diets for great masses of people such as appear in the monthly woman's magazines or the Sunday supplements. These may work for some but will fail or even prove harmful for others. But for the student of Yoga the principles outlined above should present a fairly comprehensive guide and if he will observe the effects of various foods and their combinations upon himself he will soon develop a sensible and rewarding program in keeping with his Yoga study. Also, one who frequents a health-food store will have access to additional literature which will aid in developing his knowledge of foods and their properties. Continue to perform your own tests and experiments and you will gradually find the path most suitable for *you*. If you are under the care of a physician always consult him regarding your diet. I would like to interject here that the student of Yoga who is truly interested in retaining the characteristics of youth should resort to the use of more natural products in his hygiene. That is, there are soaps, toothpastes and cosmetics for all needs that are made from natural elements and have a minimum of chemicals. Such products are becoming more well known and more widely distributed. A health-food store is probably still the best source of such products, although I would like to refer our women readers to the finer cosmetic stores which are beginning to carry the natural cosmetic lines. Honey and almond creams, fruit creams, papaya toothpaste, olive oil soaps are examples of natural products highly suitable for both men and women.

It must be obvious that there is great vital force discharged during sexual intercourse. It is to retain this vital force that Yogis, who correspond to what we in the Western world know as monks and nuns (those unmarried men and women who live an exceptionally austere life in every respect), remain celibate. It is their intention to conserve the vital force and to use it for spiritual purposes. This is one of the paths of Yoga. But there are a number of paths suitable for people in all walks of life. For the American who must be active in society the path known as *Karma* Yoga is the most practical. In this method one carries out all of the necessary activities which society requires of him, including that of sex, as necessary. It is never the intention of the *Karma* Yogi to call attention to his interest in or practice of Yoga and his dedication to self-realization. Therefore, he never allows himself to be labeled as "odd," "strange," or other adjectives which people are quick to apply to anyone who does not conform to what is supposed to be the "norm." The Yogi's self-realization work takes place inwardly and perhaps only a few intimates are aware of his practice. What we suggest to the aspiring American Yogi with regard to sex is that he follow his natural biological cycles (which are rhythmic and periodic) and not allow himself to remain in a state of perpetual sexual excitation through the artificial stimuli which the mediums of entertainment and advertising inspire. Since one is continually confronted with every possible suggestion of sex wherever he turns it is difficult to realize that most of his sexual desires are cerebral, i.e., much more a state of mind than a true need of the body. Once this is truly understood, a great deal of this mental agitation is relieved and a tremendous amount of energy which is tied up with it is released.

Let us summarize this discussion of the ability to retain and quickly replace vital elements as follows: nature and its agent the vital force are always working for you, to keep you healthy, fit, youthful and alive and to give you a continual sense of well-being both in body and in mind. All nature asks of you is that you listen to her and trust her. Therefore, the student of Yoga should attempt in all aspects of his life to revert more and more to everything which he senses is natural. He should eat more natural foods in simple combinations. He should eat when he is hungry, not when the clock tells him to do so. He should rest or sleep when his body tells him to do so. He should seek fresh air and pure water. He should attempt to get in tune with the natural biological rhythms of his organism and allow the wisdom of his body to instruct him in its care. The body is very wise, and as the vital force increases your body will tell you what it needs and will direct you to the elements which contain

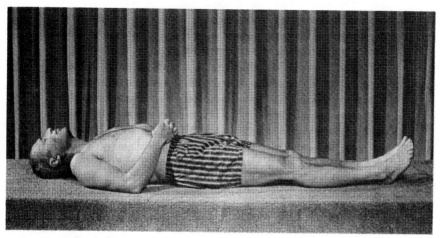

Fig. 51

Fig. 52

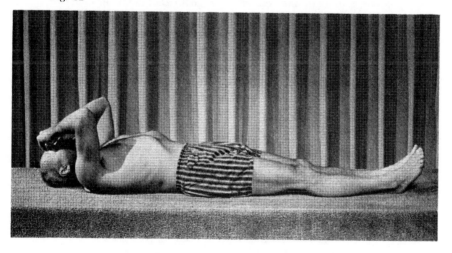

these necessities. This is a wonderful accomplishment because you will find that you are relieved of many worries regarding your health. *The more natural your life, the more you must radiate youth and all of its characteristics.*

Finally, I would like to offer you a truly remarkable technique, which is one of the most dynamic methods for restoring and increasing the vital force and all of its manifestations. This technique does not form part of the regular course but is to be used whenever necessary to replenish the vital force. Because this must be classified as a metaphysical technique we cannot offer data which will make its use valid to the physiologist or scientist; but the fact that it has such remarkable and immediate effects in revitalization and has been used for thousands of years by the Yogi for this purpose should make it sufficiently intriguing for every reader to attempt.

We will refer to this technique as "The Direction of the Vital Force." What we will be doing in essence is consciously directing the revitalizing and healing power of the vital force, which we are gaining through our exercises, to areas of the body where such energy may be needed. The procedure is this: we will use our fingers to contact an area where a great amount of vital force is stored; this center is the *solar plexus*. Next, we will draw the vital force from the solar plexus into the fingertips. Finally, we will transfer the fingertips to the head and flood the entire head with the vital force. Here is the exact method:

1. Lie on your back. Lower your eyelids. Relax completely.

2. Place the fingertips of both hands on your solar plexus. The solar plexus is that delicate area at the top of the abdomen, sometimes referred to as the "pit of the stomach." (Fig. 51)

3. Exhale through the nose and begin to take a slow COM-PLETE BREATH but do not make the movements exaggerated and do not raise your shoulders. Now as you take the slow COMPLETE BREATH, attempt to visualize a

bright white light flowing in through your nose, going down into the solar plexus and being drawn into your fingertips. The white light is the vital force. It is present whether or not you can visualize it but if you will attempt to see it you will make the technique more dynamic.

4. Retain the breath in your lungs for several seconds while you gently transfer your fingertips to the center of your forehead.

5. Exhale slowly and visualize the vital force, in the form of the white light flooding your entire head. (Fig. 52)

6. When the exhalation is completed, transfer your fingertips back to the solar plexus and repeat.

Comments: to obtain the greatest benefits this exercise should be done in groups of 21 repetitions, since it requires time to have the energies flow as desired. It may be difficult to visualize the white light; you may catch glimpses of it from time to time and then it will fade away. If this is the case, attempt to bring it back as often as possible. If you cannot visualize it at all, this will not necessarily impede the benefits to be derived from the technique. But at all times, attempt to keep your mind on what you are doing and know that you are doing this for replenishment and revitalization. The results will be self-evident. Whenever necessary, the vital force can be directed to any part of the body which is tense, tired, strained or pained. For example, if a shoulder is tense, the fingertips will be directed from the solar plexus during the inhalation to the shoulder during the exhalation; if there is a headache, the fingertips will be directed to the head as previously described; if there is a pain in the back you can move your fingertips around to the back during the exhalation and it will not impede the effect if the hands are separated to move around to an area of the back. (Naturally you would have to be in a seated posture if the back were being treated.) Since this technique has great healing properties, which are directed through the medium of the hands, it can be used to benefit others once you have gained some mastery of the procedure. To use it in connection with another person, the method is as follows: the inhalation is exactly as previously described; during the retention of breath the fingertips are moved to the afflicted area of the person in question; during the exhalation the vital force is visualized, in the form of the white light, if possible, flowing into the other's body. The technique must be repeated in groups of 21. After the first group of 21 there can be a pause of some minutes and then the repetition, etc. If the person whom you wish to help in any way objects to the technique, do not do it. If the person is in sympathy with this method of natural healing, he can be of aid if he will also attempt to visualize the white light flowing into his body when your fingers touch the afflicted area. Children respond particularly well to this method, especially when applied by the parent. Many students have at least partial success with this technique even upon first attempts, and most people have far more ability to direct the vital force than they realize. Don't fail to take advantage of this ancient technique for natural revitalization whenever you feel rundown or you have reached a low point in your biological cycle. You will find you have gained a powerful ally in your battle against the characteristics of age.

Here is the routine to be emphasized for:

REPLACEMENT OF VITAL ELEMENTS

Re-read the information on page 162

This routine can be performed at any time of the day for the above purposes.

Preliminary Leg pull	(1)
Chest Expansion	(7)
Cobra	(8)
Complete Breath	(10)
Shoulder Stand or Head Stand	(11, 20)
Direction of the vital force	(Chapter 7)

8. THE YOUTHFUL MIND

<table>
<tr><td align="center">*YOUTH*</td><td align="center">*AGE*</td></tr>
<tr><td>Alertness and clarity of the faculties of mind; optimism.</td><td>Weakening of the faculties of mind resulting in senility; depression.</td></tr>
</table>

There are two aspects of the "Youthful Mind" to consider in this discussion. The first is the prevention of a weakening of the faculties of mind and the maintenance of alertness and clarity. This we seek to accomplish through the physical exercises, the most important of which (for the brain) have been discussed in connection with blood circulation. Most of the signs of age which we have investigated in this book are obvious physical characteristics. That is, you do not have to be exceptionally perceptive to know that you are overweight, that you have lost your muscle tone or that you are stiff, inflexible, etc. But it is often difficult to be aware of the gradual loss of alertness, memory and other thought processes. These are things that usually do not become evident either to yourself or to others until they are serious. So we must make every effort to *prevent* a loss of these qualities through proper Yoga practice and good nutrition. The Yogi does not assume that there must be a loss of the faculties of mind simply because one grows older in years.

All exercises which bring an increased supply of blood into the upper areas of the body are excellent for maintenance of alertness and clarity. In the HEAD STAND, SHOULDER STAND, LOCUST, CHEST EXPANSION, COMPLETE BREATH and ALTERNATE NOSTRIL BREATHING there is increased nourishment for the brain cells. The HEAD STAND is particularly dynamic for activating these cells and the Yogis believe that there is a definite stimulation and awakening of a part of the brain which is generally dormant or functions only partially. You can imagine the increase in perception and thought power if a part of the brain which had been dormant was gradually activated. The curious part of this is that most students of Yoga sense instinctively that there *is* great potential brain power available to them! The publicity given the HEAD STAND in connection with Yoga (so much so that for years I had to explain to people that Yoga meant more than standing on the head) is justified, not as a peculiarity but as a tremendously dynamic technique that has the most marvelous effect on the brain. Make every attempt to perfect the HEAD STAND; it may take time but it is well worth your efforts. We are never in a hurry to attain the extreme position of any of the postures; our concept is always little-by-little. If you feel that you are having no success in your attempts with the HEAD STAND as described in the first part of this text then you may try the following modification: lie on your bed and allow your chest, head and arms to go over the edge, as far down as possible. The arms should touch the floor for support and the head will automatically come down. This is a very modified position but is certainly better than no inversion at all and may prove helpful for elderly people or those who find the regular HEAD STAND is strenuous for the neck.

When the brain functions well there is a general feeling of alertness, well-being and brightness. These result in optimism and optimism is usually synonymous with a sense of humor. There are no more positive attributes of youth than optimism and a sense of humor, and their opposites—pessimism, loss of hope, lack of humor—are certainly characteristics of age. You cannot fake optimism: you must have a real feeling of well-being to radiate true optimism. The above-named exercises, which emphasize good blood circulation, especially in the brain, will help to promote exhilaration and optimism.

The second aspect of the "Youthful Mind" is more abstract. We are now concerned with what can be considered a paradox, for in order to have a youthful mind one must possess a *mature* mind. A youthful mind is one which has matured to the point where it remains perpetually *open*. It does not shut down at a certain time of life and tenaciously cling to patterns which it has developed from limited ideas, thoughts and events. "Closing" is characteristic of an *old* mind, a mind which is stagnant and lifeless. A person who is twenty years old can have an old mind. The youthful mind remains young by continually rebuilding and developing itself through the nourishment of new ideas. It is not afraid to seek new concepts and surrender old ones. How is such a state of mind reached? Here, the infinite wisdom of the mental and philosophical aspects of Yoga (particularly *Raja* Yoga) can be appreciated. It is not the intention of Yoga to make people alike. On the contrary, it is the objective of Yoga to stress the complete and utter individuality of each person and have him achieve his own and unique self-expression. But here a curious paradox occurs, for in the process of gaining the freedom which is a result of genuine self-expression, the student of Yoga realizes that this can materialize only if he reaches that which is the *common source of self-expression for all persons!* If he is not aware of this source and cannot contact it he cannot be himself; he cannot realize his own true nature. He will thus act only in accordance with lifeless ideas that are imposed upon him from the outside. He will go through the motions of life but he cannot be truly alive because he has not found his own center. Therefore he acts and lives without imagination, originality or creativity.

At this point a definition of the word "Yoga" is in order. "Yoga" means *integration*. When one begins to contact the source of his existence he automatically integrates himself with this source. Then his individuality and uniqueness must shine through. True self-expression means forever becoming, and is eternally new. Again, this is not a forced attempt to be original or creative (which can never be more than imitative), but a spontaneous event in which one joyously becomes the medium, or sounding board, for the expressions of the Absolute, God, the source of his existence. When this happens, the individual is freed from the terribly confining limitations of what he has heretofore conceived of as "me" or "I," and the necessity of protecting the phantom which is known as the "Ego." The energy released from the carrying of this burden is tremendous and the ego dissolves to the degree in which the seeker opens himself to the expressions of the Absolute. In this state of consciousness, one is no longer concerned with keeping up with the Joneses (in all levels of society and in all fields of endeavor); he is always ahead of them by mere virtue of the fact that he is *himself*. He is distinct and unique and nothing can be like him. He is at last completely and truly secure and at rest in this knowledge.

The practice of meditation is a practice in which the Yogi concentrates on contacting the Absolute. Meditation was discussed briefly in the instructions regarding the LOTUS postures. In the serious practice of meditation the Yogi attempts consciously to open himself more and more to the expressions of the Absolute. This can be done actively or passively. That is, one can attempt to contact his true nature during his everyday activities, in the midst of his work. This is particularly applicable to people engaged in work requiring some creativity. Artists, writers, musicians, architects, designers, etc., are instinctively seeking to have closer and closer contact with their center; but there is no situation in which any person cannot attempt this contact. *It requires only the desire to do so.*

Passive meditation is the classical form of contacting the Absolute. The method is one of the simplest procedures man can undertake, the effects, the most profound. Let us learn the method of passive meditation. The procedure consists of secluding yourself in a quiet, pleasant place once or twice each day (perhaps following your Yoga practice) and sitting in the LOTUS or CROSS-LEGGED posture. Next, concentrate on your breathing. Attempt to breathe so quietly that you cannot hear the breath as it is inhaled and exhaled and until you breathe so slowly that you are breathing no more than about 3 times per minute. You breathe deeply with the lower and upper areas of the lungs but with an absolute minimum of bodily movement. The more you are able to slow down your breathing the less disturbed your mind will be. The more quiet your mind becomes the more contact it is possible to make with your center. You do not have to think about what you are doing or that you are attempting to accomplish something. All that is necessary is to become as completely still both in body and mind as is possible. Sitting in the LOTUS will quiet the body. Breathing very slowly and silently will begin to quiet the mind. To keep the mind from continually wandering it is a traditional practice to count your breaths. Begin with one and count to ten. Then repeat, never going beyond ten. When you find your mind wandering, bring it back to the counting. Do not grow impatient with the mind for being distracted; simply continue to bring it gently back to your counting of the breaths. Sit absolutely motionless. The moment you grow uncomfortable or move for any reason whatsoever your meditation for that period is over. This should be approximately 10 minutes to begin with and gradually be extended.

The Absolute is always ready to reveal itself and relieve you of the great burden of the ego if you can become sufficiently quiet and passive to permit it to do so. The classical example is the pool of clear water. Regardless of the purity and clarity of the water, if the surface is disturbed with ripples you cannot see through to the bottom. When the ripples are stilled and the surface becomes quiet the bottom can be clearly seen. The pool represents the Absolute and the ripples are the continual thoughts and agitation of the mind which perpetuates the ego. The gradual contact gained through the patient practice of passive meditation will carry over into all of your activities. Once this contact is made and sustained the mind can never grow old but remains in a state of constant renewal because it is in tune with the source of life itself. And so, what may very well be the most significant of all of the characteristics of youth, the Youthful Mind, is within the reach of all students of Yoga.

Here is the routine to be emphasized for:

ALERTNESS AND CLARITY

Re-read the information on page 162

This routine can be performed at any time of the day for the above purpose.

Chest Expansion	(7)
Complete Breath	(10)
Shoulder Stand or Head Stand	(11, 20)
Alternate Nostril Breathing	(14)
Locust	(15)
Meditation (Chapter 8)	

Abdomen:
    Alternate Leg Pull for reducing, 126-129
    Locust strengthens, 112
    Plough for strengthening, 130-34
    preventing flabbiness, 126-219
    reducing weight, 116
    reducing weight and firming skin, 130-134
    Toe Twist aids in streamlining, 44-47
    Yoga exercises for muscle tone, 193
Abdominal Contraction, for muscle tone, 190
Abdominal Lift, 98-101
    how to perform, 98-99
    how to practice, 100
    to improve quality of blood, 187
    for muscle tone, 190
"Age and aging,"
    cause and solution for, 8-9
    characteristics of, 5-6
    problems of, 4
    real meaning of youth and, 4-6
    symptoms of, 8, 186
        due to improper care of body, 9-10
    wrong approach to the problems of, 6-8
Air, source of vital force, 203-205
Alcoholic beverages, use of, 207, 210
Alertness of mind, Yoga techniques for, 6, 225
Alternate Leg Pull, 126-129, 161
    how to perform, 126-127
    how to practice, 128-129
Alternate Nostril Breathing, 102-105
    how to perform, 102-104
    how to practice, 104
Americans, importance of Yoga for, 11-12

Ankles:
    Full-Lotus for elasticity of, 55
    Half-Lotus releases tension in, 52-54
Anxiety, 164-166
    Alternate Nostril Breathing to relieve, 102-105
    postures for overcoming, 57
Appearance, Complete Breath aids in improving, 78
Arm and Leg Stretch, 161
    how to perform, 48-50
    how to practice, 50-51
    objectives, 48, 50
    for releasing trapped energy, 48-51
    for relief from tension and fatigue, 93
    time allowance, 50
Arms:
    Arm and Leg Stretch, 48-51
    exercises to improve muscle tone, 191, 193
    Locust develops and strengthens, 112
    Yoga exercises for muscle tone, 193
    Yoga exercises to reduce, 199
Arthritis, Yoga exercises for, 157
Arthritis National Research Foundation, 157n
Atrophication, not inevitable, 10
Auto-suggestion, 167
Awareness, developing sense of, 204
Back (See also Spine)
    Alternate Leg Pull for developing shoulders and, 126-129
    Bow stretches back, 116-119
    Cobra technique for, 66-69
    developing elasticity of the spine, 140-142
    developing lumbar and shoulder areas, 126-129

LaVergne, TN USA
20 December 2010
209532LV00003B/3/P